Cooking My Way

From Sunrise to Sunset
Cheap Nutritious Food

Helen Thomas

First published 2017
Publisher DH & EH Grugeon
6 Tralee St, Bracken Ridge, Queensland, 4017 Australia

© Helen Thomas 2017
The moral rights of the author have been asserted

National Library of Australia Cataloguing-in-Publication entry

Creator: Thomas, Helen, 1946- author.

Title: Cooking my way: from sunrise to sunset - cheap nutritious food / Helen Thomas.

ISBN: 9781925319057 (paperback)
ISBN 9781925319064 (Epub)

Subjects: Low budget cooking.
Cooking.
Nutrition.

All rights reserved. Except as permitted under the *Australian Copyright Act* 1968 (for example a fair dealing for the purposes of study, research, criticism or review), no part of this book may be reproduced, stored in a retrieval system, communicated, or transmitted in any form or by any means without prior written permission. All enquiries should be made to the publisher at the address above.

Disclaimer

The material in this book is of the nature of general information only. The information in this book is not intended to be taken as medical advice or to indicate the suitability of particular foods in any specific circumstances. The publisher and author expressly disclaim any liability to any person because of any action taken or not taken in reliance, in whole or in part, on the content of this publication. If you have medical issues, you should consult a qualified medical practitioner.

Drink at least 2 litres (4 pints) of water each day

Contents

Introduction 1
Breakfast 2
Lunch 2
Soup 3
    Pumpkin Soup 4
    Tomato, Carrot and Basil Soup 5
    Helen's Winter Soup 6
    Leek, Potato, Corn and Parsley Soup 7
    Lentils, Potato, Mushroom and Onion Soup 8
Fish 9
    Marinara (Seafood Mix) with Pasta 10
    Fish Pie 11
    Fish Curry 12
Chicken 13
    Chicken Wings 14
    Chicken Curry (Mild) 15
    Chicken with Vegetables and Noodles 16
Beef 17
    Beef Curry 18
    Shepherd's Pie 19
    Spaghetti Bolognaise 20
Pork 21
    Belly of Pork and Pineapple Curry 22
    Belly of pork strips with mashed potato, steamed vegetables, and a side salad 23
    Pork chop, baked potato, and steamed vegetables 24
Lamb 25
    Lamb or Oxtail Stew 26
    Moussaka 27
Vegetables 29
    Yellow Potato in Turmeric & Coconut Sauce 30
    Devilled Potato 31
    Mashed Potato 32
    Roast Vegetables 33
    Steamed Vegetables 34
    Vegetable bake with cheese 35
    Lentils with Spinach 36

Salads	37
Coleslaw	38
Potato Salad with Hard-boiled Eggs and Chives	39
Raw Vegetable Salad	40
Eggplant Salad	41
Colourful Salad	42
Rice	43
About Rice	43
Yellow Rice	45
Stir Fried Rice and Vegetables	46
Growing time	47
Curry Leaf (Murraya koenigii)	47
Lemon Grass (Cymbopogon citratus)	47
Pandanus leaf (Pandanus latifolius, P. amaryllifolius)	47
Last Words	48

Introduction

Dear Readers

Thank you for taking the time to buy, read and try cooking the recipes in my book.

I have been very concerned that so many people throughout the world are finding that they do not have enough money to put food on the table.

I have done a lot of research and found that cooking cheaply and nutritiously should be within almost everyone's financial reach.

In this book, I concentrate on providing some basic recipes that use cheap ingredients, that are lovely to eat, and that are full of good nutrition. I also include some cooking tips to get the best value for your shopping money.

I am also very concerned at the number of people I see who are overweight or very obese. This is a plague that is seriously affecting the health of people in developed countries and is why I am concentrating on healthy nutritious food.

Remember to drink 2 litres (4 pints) of water to be able to flush your kidneys and to keep you hydrated.

Please remember your portion control, and don't forget to drink your water. Try to exercise as often as you can. Walking is very good for all of us to do, so try to go for a walk with other people so that you keep safe. If it is possible, try to get together with other people who live in the neighbourhood and make up a walking group. Happy walking and happy exercising.

I will be writing a recipe book every two months. My next cookery book will be out at the beginning of October 2017. I will have the Christmas cookery book out at the beginning of November. This will cover November and December 2017.

I would love to hear from you and learn what you think of my recipes, what you eat as your main food and what recipes you would like me to include in future books. If we are in touch, I will be able to let you know when books are released. Please get in touch with me at helen.thomas@wise.works and see my website at CookingWithFewIngredients.com.

Best regards and enjoy my recipes

Helen Thomas

Breakfast

I usually have a high protein breakfast. I have two soft boiled eggs, a slice of bread (toasted)a dash of butter or margarine, salt and pepper, with a banana. That is my usual breakfast during the week. Sometimes we have a small amount of cooked breakfast at the weekend.

A high protein breakfast keeps you full until midday. I have a piece of fruit as a mid-morning snack.

Lunch

We can have a sandwich of salad and cold meat, I sometimes make a quick meal with noodles and whatever vegetables I have in the fridge.

Remember your portion control

If you can, have hard boiled eggs, or sliced chicken or turkey. Try to eat a variety of green vegetables.

Please remember to drink 2 litres (over 4 pints) of water a day to flush out your kidneys, keep you healthy and assist weight control.

Soup

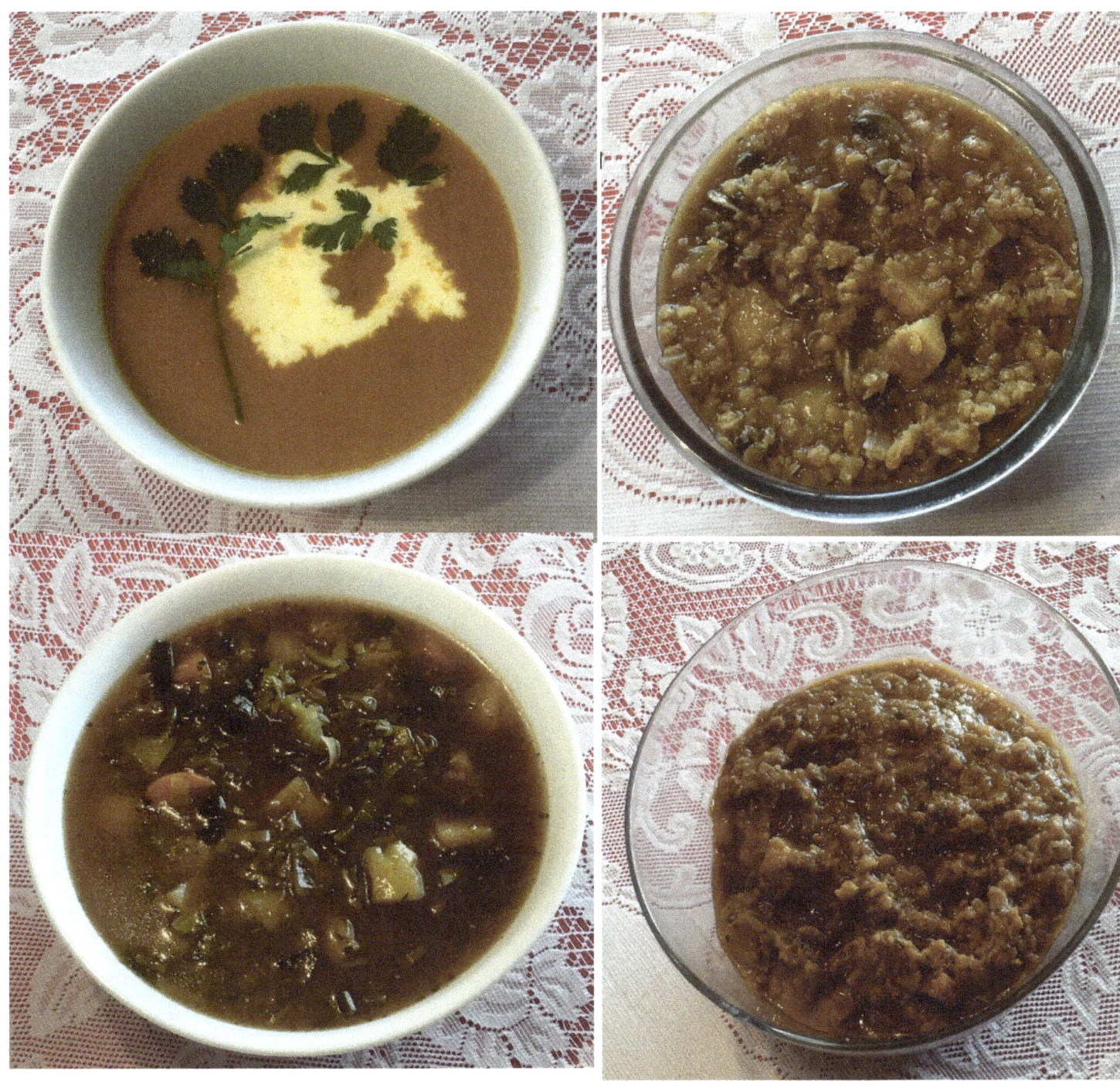

Pumpkin Soup

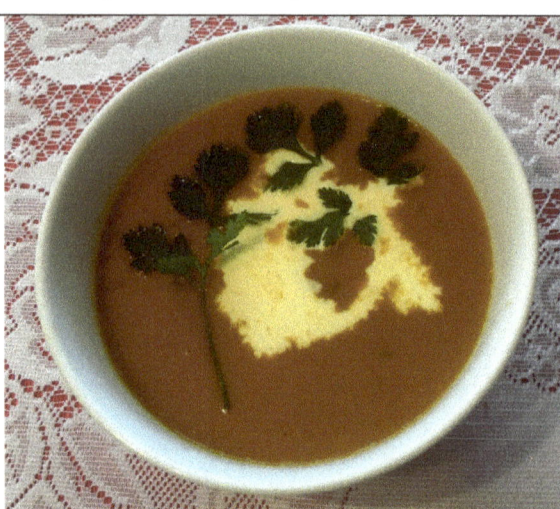

Ingredients (serves 4)

400g (12oz) Pumpkin
½ bunch Coriander (Cilantro)
Oil for frying
1 large onion
1 tsp crushed garlic
½ litre (I Pt) Chicken or vegetable stock
Pepper and salt to taste

Method

Peel pumpkin and cut into 1cm (1/2 in) cubes
Wash Coriander thoroughly, remove roots and chop roughly.
Chop onion
Fry onion and garlic gently until onion is translucent
Add pumpkin and fry until lightly browned
Add coriander and stock and bring to boil
Reduce heat and simmer until pumpkin is well cooked (about 20 minutes)
Liquidise in a liquidiser, food processor, or with an electric stick blender.
Taste and season with freshly ground black pepper and salt.
Bring back to the boil and simmer for 5 minutes. Stir well.

Tips

You can stir in a swirl of plain yoghurt
Eat slowly, so you enjoy your food.
Remember your portion control

Portion Control

I find that limiting my portion sizes is essential to maintaining a reasonable weight. The stomach is, naturally, only a little larger than a tennis ball. It can expand when more food is stuffed into it, and that is what gives us that overfull feeling and makes us lethargic.

It takes about 20 minutes from eating for us to feel full. For this reason, we need to eat slowly and allow time for the full feeling to develop. Eating a *small* snack fifteen or twenty minutes before we have our meal, helps the stomach not to feel empty so we can avoid that ravenous feeling.

Tomato, Carrot and Basil Soup

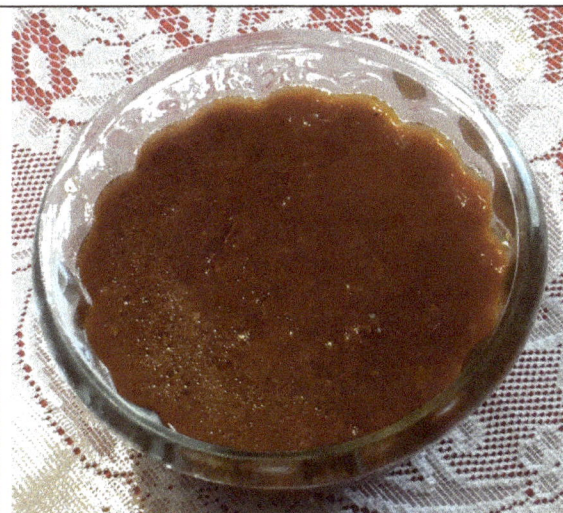

Ingredients (serves 4)

1 large onion
A dash of cooking oil
500 g (1 lb) ripe tomatoes
500 g (1 lb) carrots
1 bunch basil
Salt to taste
Black pepper
A dash of Worcestershire sauce
1 carton vegetable stock
Pepper and salt to taste

Method
Slice onion, Fry in oil
Add salt and pepper
Cut tomatoes into cubes
Cut carrots into small cubes
Add tomatoes and carrots to onions and stir
Add the vegetable stock
Let it cook on a low heat for 20-30 minutes
Chop basil and add it to the soup at the last minute
Let it cool for about 15 minutes
Liquidise the soup in a liquidiser or with an electric stick mixer
.

Tips
If you wish you could have a dash of cream and some shredded basil on top of each bowl of soup
Eat slowly, so you enjoy your food.
Remember your portion control

Helen's Winter Soup

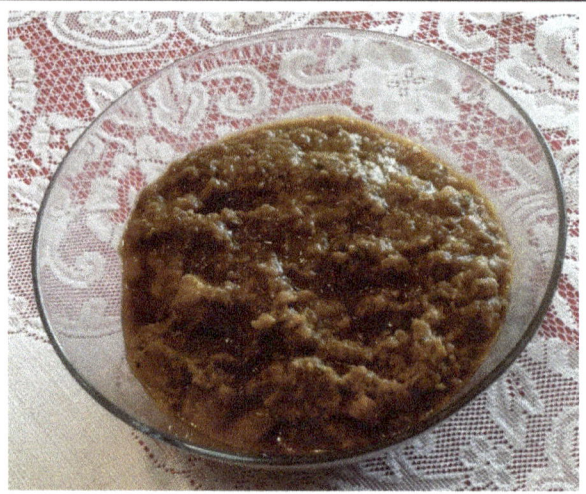

Ingredients (serves 4)

2 large potatoes
2 large onions
2 tbsp oil
2 cups red lentils
2 large carrots
2 sticks celery with leaves on
2 tbsp Worcestershire sauce
2 tbsp soy sauce
3 or 4 litres (3 to 4 qts) vegetable stock
Dash of garlic paste
Dash of ginger paste
3 heaped tbsp miso paste

Method
Slice the onions and fry in a large saucepan.
Wash lentils until the water runs clear. Add to onions
Wash, peel and dice the potatoes
Cut carrots and celery. Add potatoes, carrots and celery to the pan. Stir well.
Add Worcestershire sauce. soy sauce, garlic, ginger and miso paste. Stir well
Be careful how much salt you add, because the miso paste, soy and Worcestershire sauces and the stock are all salty. Try to get low salt stock.
Add the stock. Bring to the boil, then lower the heat and simmer until the vegetables and lentils are cooked.
Liquidise if desired.

Tips
Serve with garlic bread, toast or bread rolls.
Eat slowly, so you enjoy your food.
Remember your portion control

This soul will keep for a few days in the fridge, or you can freeze it.

This is a wonderful soup. You can have it crunchy or, if you prefer a smooth soup, use a liquidiser or electric stick mixer.

Leek, Potato, Corn and Parsley Soup

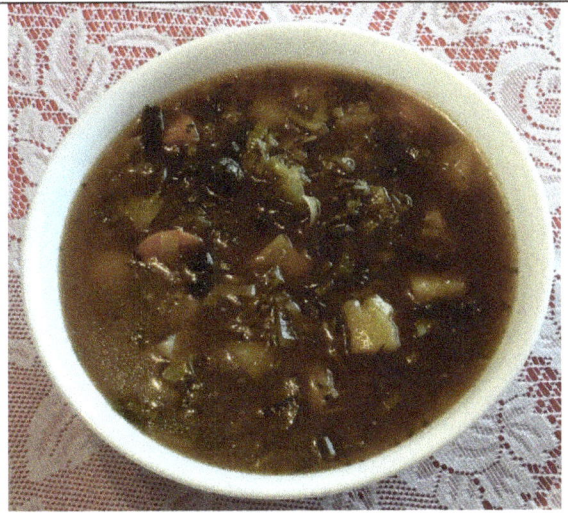

Ingredients (serves 4)

2 large leeks
2 large onions
3 large potatoes
A bunch of parsley
2 litres (4 pints) vegetable stock
1 tin corn kernels
Dash of Worcestershire sauce
Dash of soy sauce
2 tbsp Miso paste
100ml (½cup) cooking oil
Dash of garlic paste
Dash of ginger paste

Method
Chop the leeks (all of it) and wash it thoroughly as there might be sand or soil between the leaves
Slice the onions and start frying in the oil in a large pan
Wash and scrub the potatoes thoroughly. Dice and add to the onions. Stir well
Add the leeks and fry.
Rinse corn in cold water and drain. Add to pan. Stir.
Add the Worcestershire sauce, soy sauce, miso paste, vegetable stock, garlic and ginger.
Bring back to the boil then lower heat and simmer until potatoes are cooked
Wash, dry and chop the parsley and add to the soup

This can be eaten as a chunky soup, or you can use your liquidiser or electric stick mixer to puree it.

Tips
Serve with garlic bread or toast.
Eat slowly, so you enjoy your food.
Remember your portion control

Lentils, Potato, Mushroom and Onion Soup

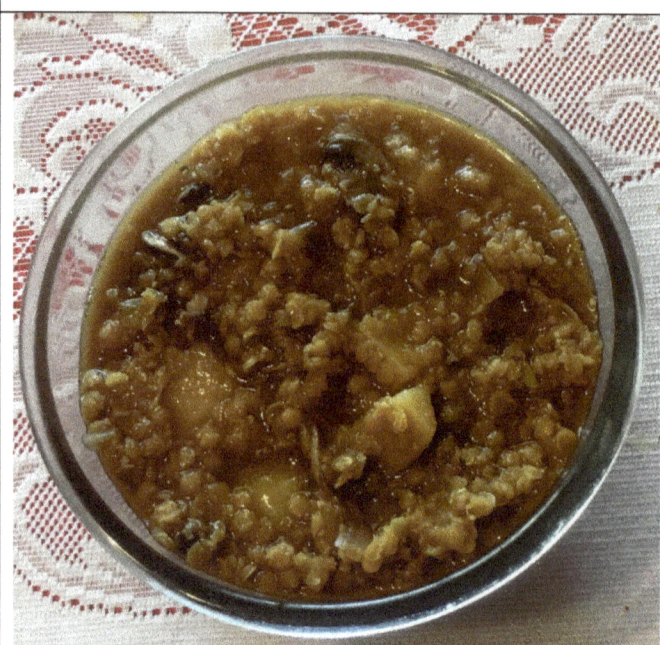

Ingredients (serves 4)

6 Large onions
2 heaped Tbsp oil
500g (1 lb) firm mushrooms
1 cup Red lentils (washed until water runs clear)
2 large potatoes (washed and scrubbed)
Salt and pepper to taste
Dash of garlic paste
Dash of ginger paste
2 litres (4 Pints) Stock (if you use vegetable stock, vegetarians can eat this soup)
Dash Worcestershire sauce
Dash Soy Sauce
2 tbsp Miso paste

Method
.Slice the onions and fry, in a large saucepan, in the oil until soft and translucent
Add washed lentils and stir
Slice mushrooms and add to pan
Dice potatoes and add. Stir well
Add Worcestershire sauce, soy sauce, miso paste, garlic, and ginger. Stir
Add Stock. Stir well
Add salt and pepper
Bring to the boil and then lower heat to simmer.
When the potatoes are cooked, the soup will be ready. It won't take too long.

Tips
This soup can be kept in the fridge for a day or two.
Freeze any remaining soup (if there is any left!)
Serve with garlic bread or toast.
Eat slowly, so you enjoy your food.
Remember your portion control

Fish

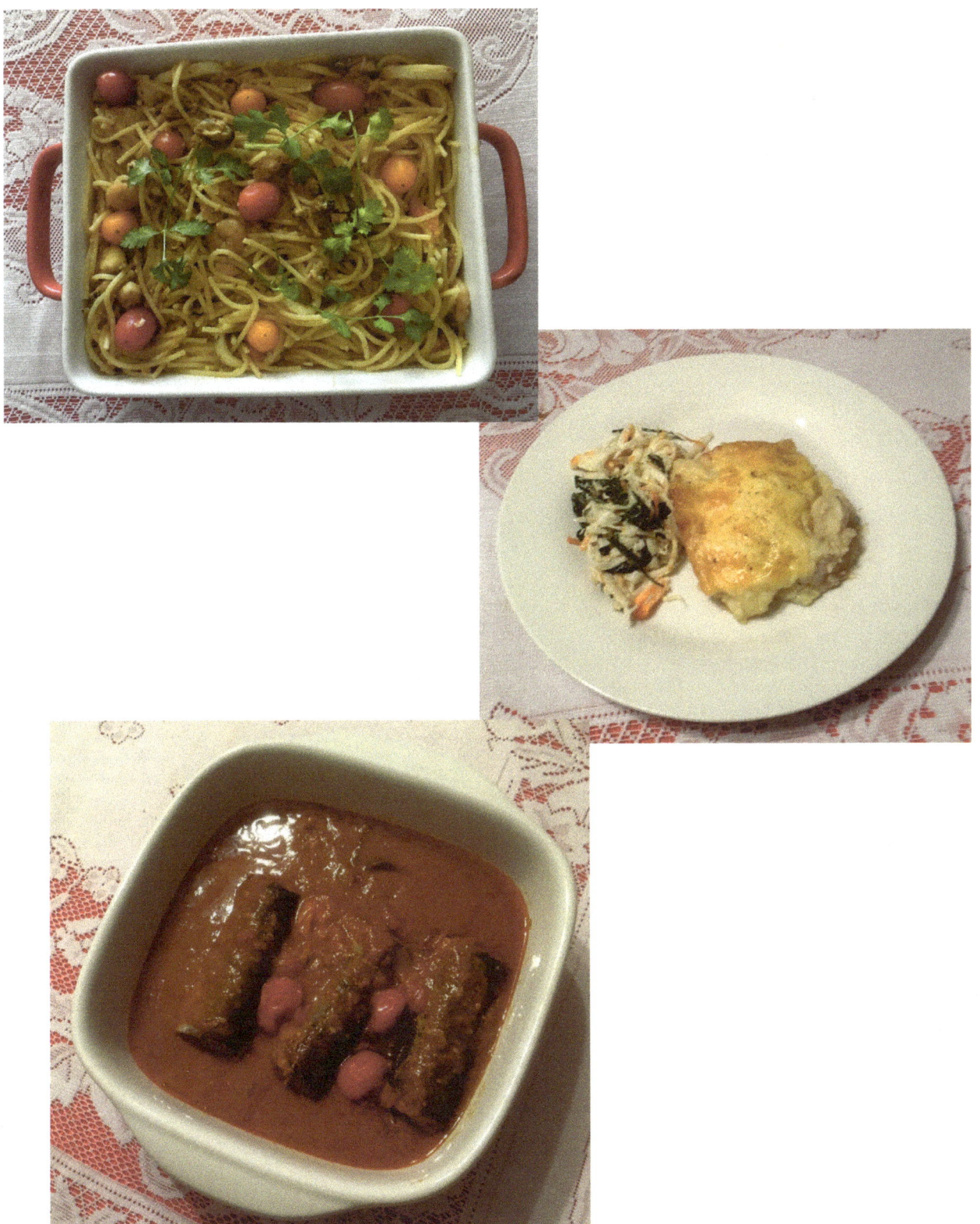

Marinara (Seafood Mix) with Pasta

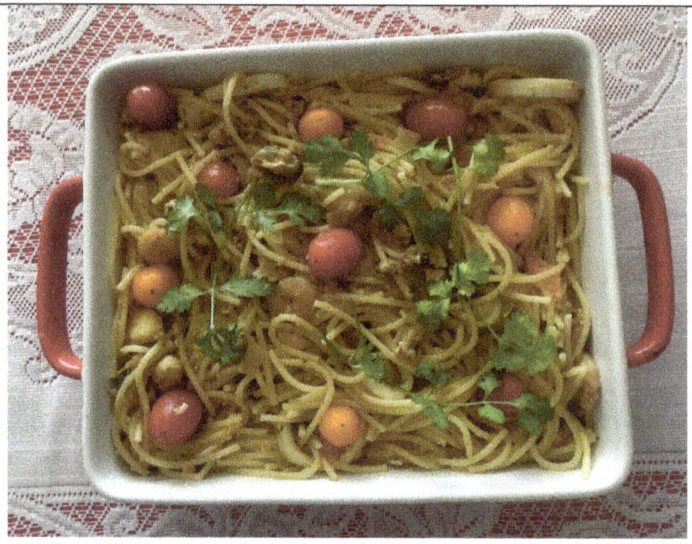

Ingredients (serves 4)

1 kg Marinara Mix (Seafood Mix)
1 large onion
Oil for frying
1 large packet macaroni (or spaghetti, broken up)
Garlic
Ginger
Paprika
Salt to taste
Coriander leaves or parsley leaves
Lemon Juice
A punnet of cherry tomatoes

Method

In a large pan, fry the sliced onion
Mix in the garlic, ginger, paprika, and salt
Cook for one minute
Stir in the marinara (seafood) mix
Cook until all the different fish is cooked, but don't overcook it.
Chop the coriander or parsley. Mix into the marinara

Meanwhile, boil a large pan filled with salted water,
Add the macaroni/spaghetti and cook until it is soft enough.
(Keep an eye on the marinara/seafood pan to ensure it does not burn or overcook)
Drain and mix into the marinara/seafood mix with the cherry tomatoes and a sprinkling of lemon juice.

Mix and serve

Tips

This meal is best eaten as soon as it is cooked
Could be topped with black pepper and grated parmesan
Serve with a side salad

Eat slowly, so you enjoy your food.
Remember your portion control

Fish Pie

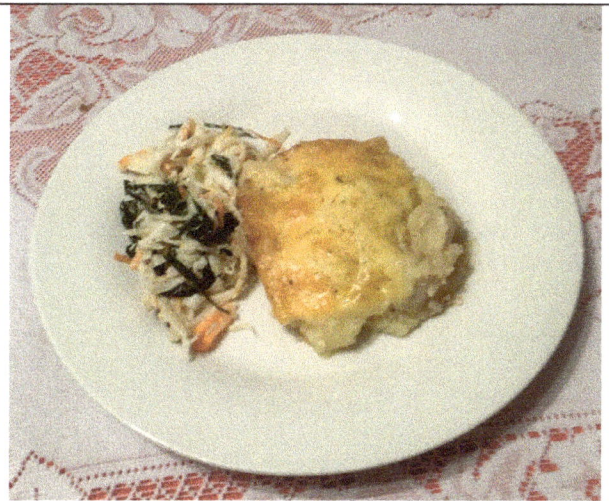

Ingredients (serves 4)

500g (1 lb) Fresh white fish or tinned fish of your choice.
Handful of cooked prawns (Optional)
1 onion sliced
1 tsp crushed Garlic or 3 cloves of garlic crushed
1 tsp minced Ginger
½ tsp dried mixed herbs
Dash of lemon juice
Salt and pepper to taste
4 cups Mashed potato (see recipe)
50 g (½ oz) Grated cheese (optional)

Method

Warm oven to 180°C 350°F
If you are going to use fresh fish, take the skin off and debone it.
Cut fish into 2cm (1 inch) squares
Fry onion until translucent in a little oil(don't burn the onions)
Add ginger, garlic, and some dried mixed herbs and cook for a few seconds
Add fish and stir
Continue cooking until fish is cooked. This will only take a few minutes.
Add prawns if you wish.
Add salt, pepper, and dash of lemon juice.
Put the fish mixture into an oven-proof dish
Arrange the potato mash on top of the fish
Sprinkle with cheese if desired
Bake for 30 to 40 minutes. Since everything is already cooked, it should not take too long to cook.

Tips

Serve with steamed vegetables

Eat slowly, so you enjoy your food.
Remember your portion control

Buy fish fillets when the cost of fish is cheaper. By doing this, you can put them in snap lock bags and freeze them so that you can use them when you wish to have a fish meal.

Fish Curry

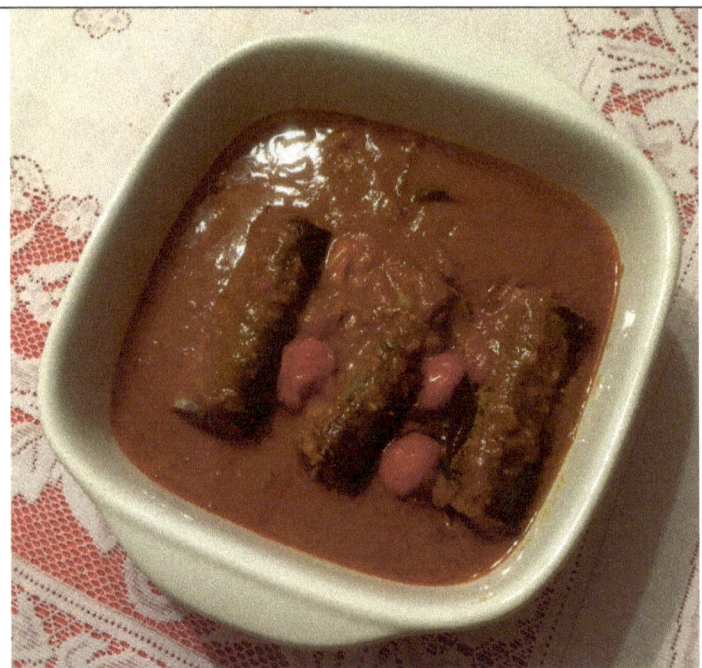

Ingredients (serves 4)

500g (1 lb) Fresh or tinned fish
I Onion sliced and fried in a little oil until soft
1 tsp crushed garlic
1 tsp crushed ginger
1 tin diced tomatoes
Fish stock
⅔ tbsp Thai red curry paste (freeze any unused)
A dash of lemon or lime juice
½ large tin of coconut milk (use the other half for lentils)
Few curry leaves
Small stem of lemon grass crushed and chopped finely
Leaf of pandanus cut up finely

Method

Slice the onion and fry over a low heat in a little oil until onion is cooked but not burned.
Add crushed garlic, ginger, and curry paste. Cook for a minute or two on a low heat.
Add chopped lemon grass, chopped pandanus and cook the sauce on a low heat.
Add the diced fish and cook for a few minutes. (If fresh fish, until the fish is cooked). Be careful not to break up the fish.

Tips
Buy fresh fish of your choice, or you can make this from tinned fish. Again, it is your choice.
It is always best if you make the sauce first and add the diced fish to the sauce for the last few minutes.
Serve with rice, stir-fried vegetables, and lentils.

Eat slowly, so you enjoy your food.
Remember your portion control

Chicken

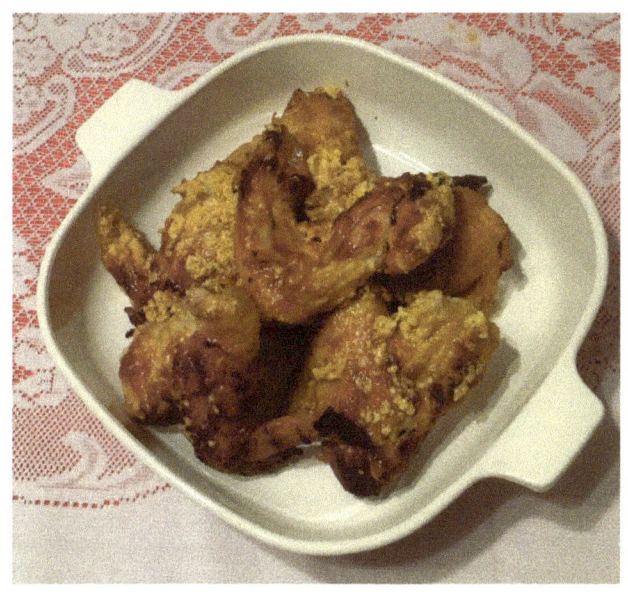

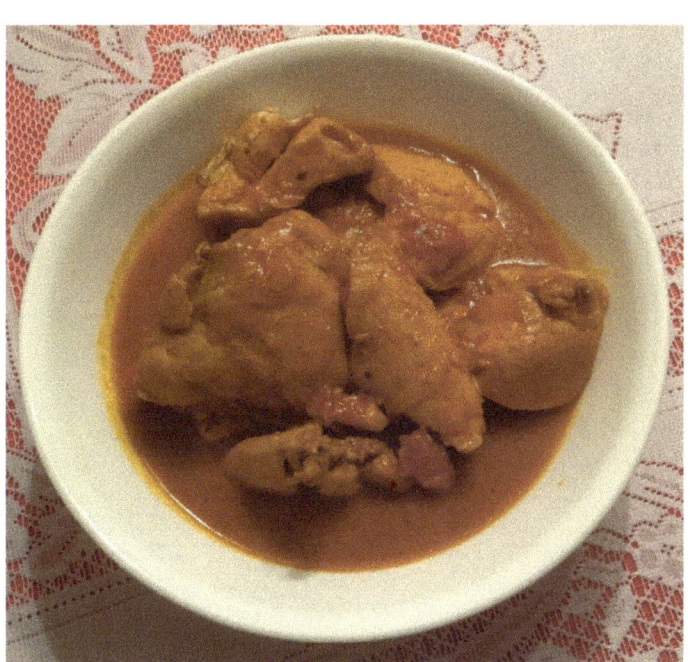

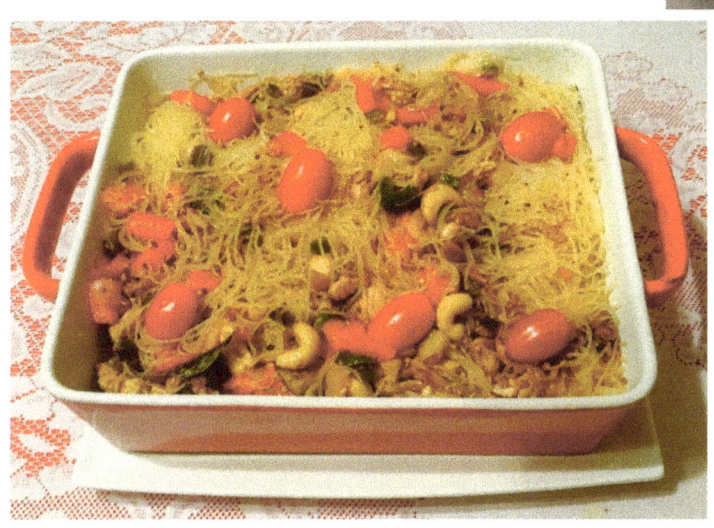

Chicken Wings

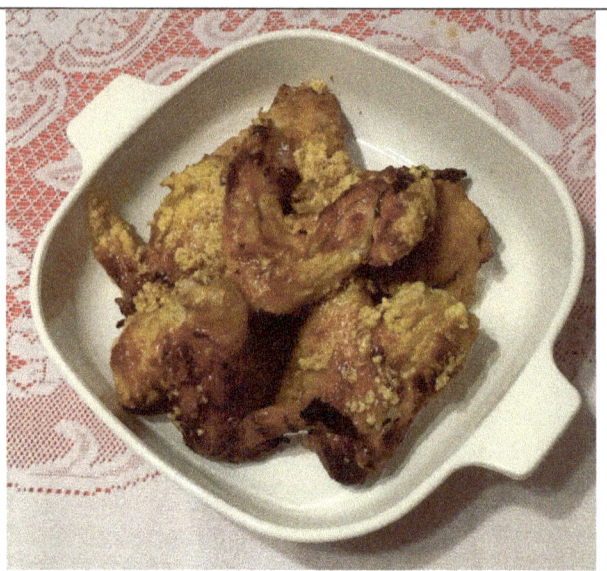

Ingredients (serves 4)

Chicken Wings according to appetite
Plain Yoghurt
Dash of Salt
1 tsp Paprika
Dash Chilli flakes(optional)
2 tbsp or to taste Curry Paste (mild)

Method

Mix some plain yoghurt, a dash of salt, a teaspoon of plain paprika, and a dash of chilli flakes (if you wish to have it a bit hot) or if you have a jar of curry paste (mild) in your cupboard, mix a bit of it into the yoghurt.
Coat the wings generously with the yoghurt mix and leave them in the fridge to marinate for at least 4 hours, or overnight.
Heat the oven to 180°C, 360°F
Arrange the coated wings on oiled foil or baking paper in a baking dish
Cook for 30 to 40 minutes. Watch the meat cooking. Turn the chicken wings after a few minutes.

Tips
Serve with steamed vegetables and mashed or jacket potato

Eat slowly, so you enjoy your food.
Remember your portion control

Chicken Curry (Mild)

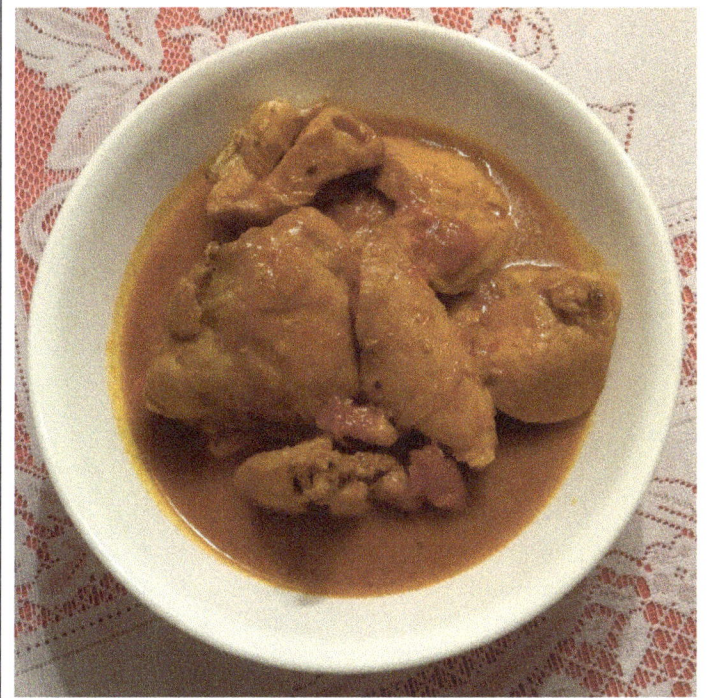

Ingredients (serves 4)

400g of chicken meat.
1 Onion or two for a whole chicken
About 2 Tbsp olive oil (or other cooking oil – Rice Bran or Sunflower oils are good)
1 generous tsp chopped ginger (I use ginger and garlic from a jar)
1 generous tsp chopped garlic
4 tbsp Curry paste (mild)
Optional (well worth using if you can get them, they really enhance the flavour – Growing instructions at the back of this book):
   2 sprigs Curry leaves (Karrapincha)
   10cm Lemon Grass (use the stems, not the green leaves) crushed
   10cm Pandanus leaf
400gm Fresh or tinned tomatoes, diced
200ml coconut milk
400ml Chicken Stock
Salt to taste

Method

If you are cooking chicken that has been frozen, make sure it is thawed completely.
Cut the chicken to suit your family, Larger chunks tend to taste better than very small ones.
Slice an onion and fry it in a little oil. Be careful not to burn the onion.
Add curry paste, garlic and ginger
If you can get them, add Curry Leaves, Lemon Grass and some Pandanus leaf. These are cooked in the curry sauce to give it flavour and then often taken out before serving. They will really enhance the flavour of the curry.
Add the chicken and fry it until brown on the outside.
Add diced tomatoes, coconut milk and stock.
Simmer, covered, until the meat is well cooked.
Season with salt.

Tips

Chicken meat – use either a whole chicken or chicken pieces. Chicken with the bone in tastes better, but chicken fillets can be used. Thigh fillets are tastier than breast fillets. I buy chicken when it is on special and freeze it.

Eat slowly, so you enjoy your food.
Remember your portion control

Chicken with Vegetables and Noodles

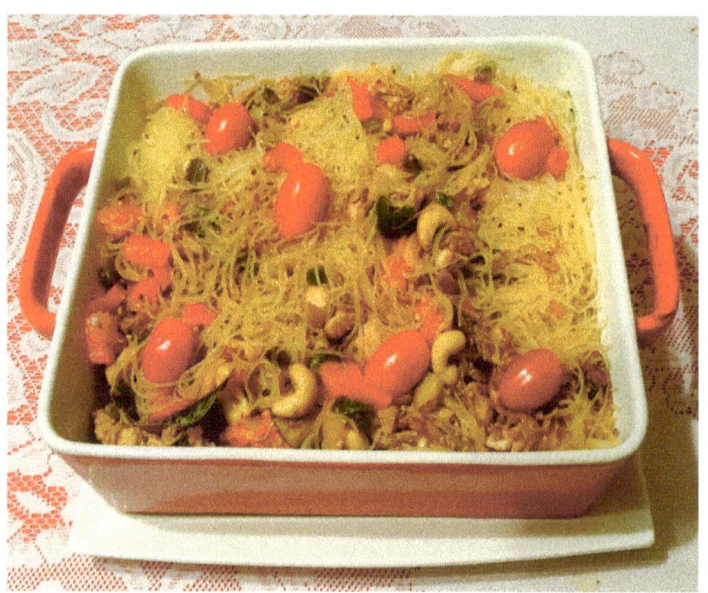

Ingredients (serves 4)

4 Squares or 250g Rice noodles
1 Large Onion
1 tsp Minced garlic
1 tsp Minced ginger
2 Tsp Sauce (Soy, Barbecue, Oyster, – whatever you have)
Salt to taste
2 Cups Diced cooked chicken (skin and bones removed) or buy a whole cooked chicken.
5 Cups Mixed vegetables (get a combination of colours)
For example:
Red/Green/Yellow peppers – diced
Zucchini (Courgette) – Diced or grated
Carrots Grated or diced and steamed
Mushrooms – Chopped – Add at last minute
Green beans – cut up and steamed

Method

Steam beans and carrots
Put rice noodles in boiling water until cooked, then drain
Dice/grate vegetables
Chop onion
Fry onion, garlic and ginger in a little oil until the onion is soft
Add chicken and fry for a minute
Add vegetables apart from mushroom and cook for about 3 minutes
Add mushrooms and cook for one minute
Add noodles and stir
Add sauce and salt to taste – go easy on the salt as some of the other ingredients will be salty. Also, do not use more than a couple of teaspoons of sauce as most sauce contains sugar and salt.
Give it a final stir.

Tips

Eat slowly, so you enjoy your food.
Remember your portion control

Beef

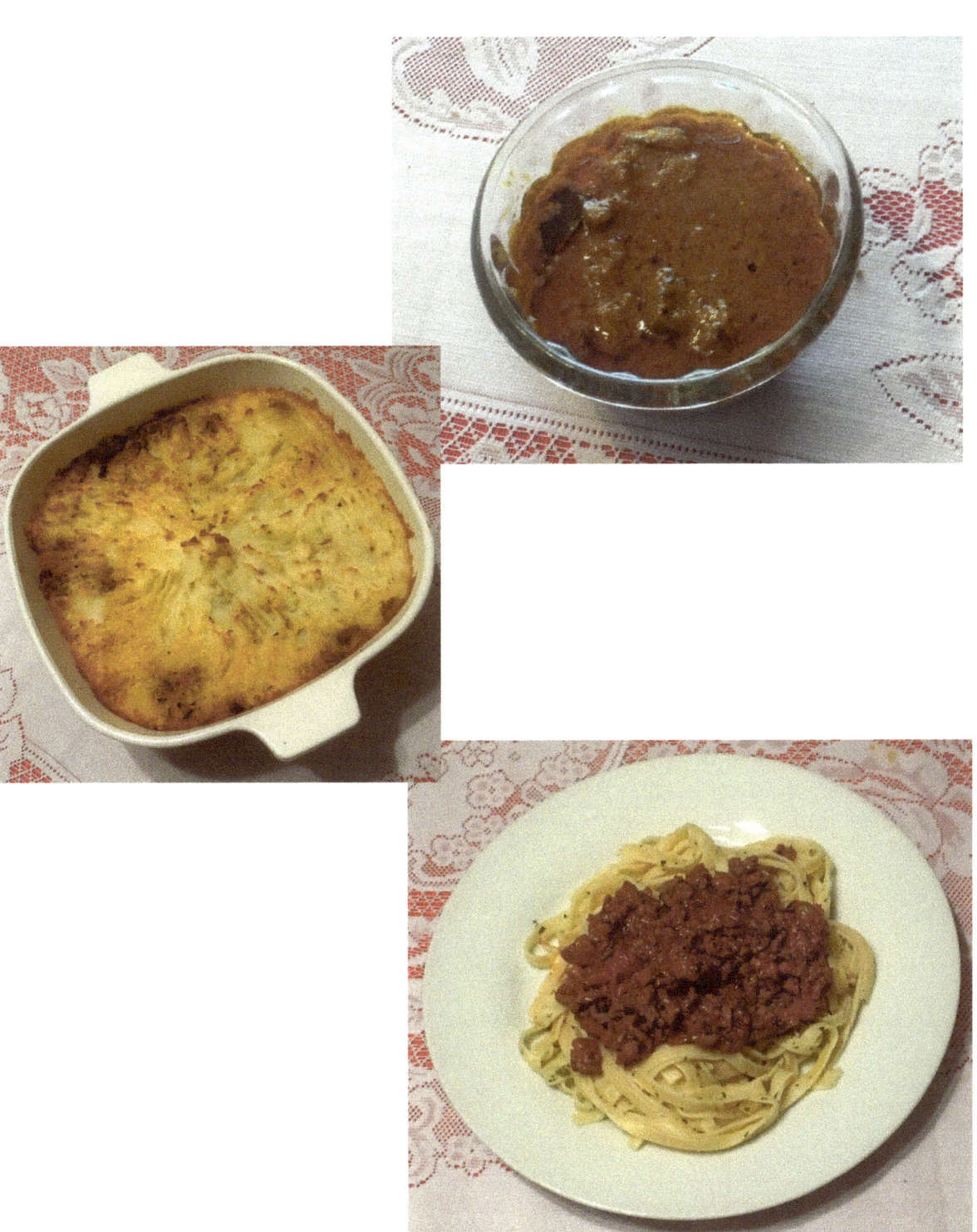

Beef Curry

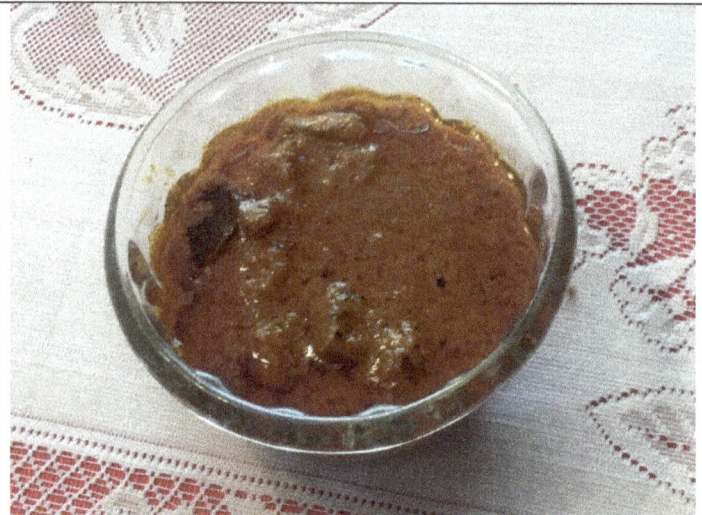

Ingredients (serves 4)

1 Kg (2 lbs) Chuck Steak or Stewing Steak
1 Large Onion
*A handful of curry leaves
*1 Small stem of lemon grass
*1 leaf of pandanus
   * If you can get them
   See p 47 for how to grow them
2 tsp garlic paste
2 tsp ginger paste
2 tbsp cooking oil
Salt to taste
3 full tbsp. curry paste (your choice)
1 tin crushed tomatoes
½ large tin coconut milk (keep the other half for another dish)
¼ to ½ a carton beef stock

Method

Cut the beef into cubes
Put the cubes on a large baking tray and bake for 20 minutes at 180 °C (360 °F)
Meanwhile, peel and slice the onion and fry in cooking oil
Add the curry leaves, lemon grass (crushed) pandanus, garlic paste, ginger paste.
Add the beef cubes and stir well
Add curry paste and tomatoes, keep stirring
Add coconut milk and beef stock
Mix well and cook on a medium to low heat until meat is cooked through.
Cover and keep stirring until curry is cooked and the meat is very tender

Tips

Serve with basmati rice, lentils, and a vegetable curry.

Eat slowly, so you enjoy your food.
Remember your portion control

Shepherd's Pie

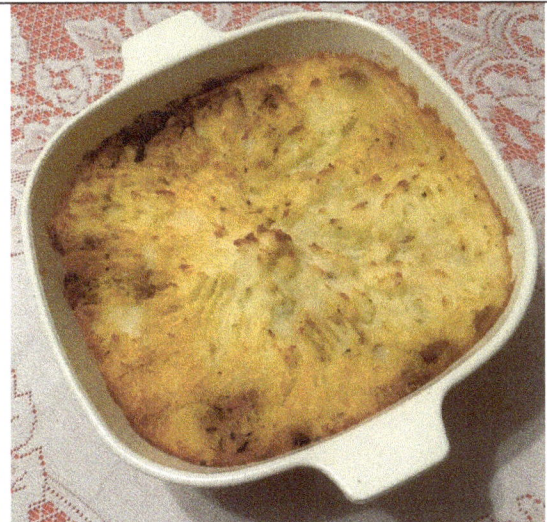

Ingredients (serves 4)

1 lb (500g) minced meat (beef or lamb)
5 medium potatoes
1 large onion
½ tsp minced or crushed garlic
½ tsp minced or crushed ginger
2 tbsp oil
1 heaped tsp dried mixed herbs
2 carrots
Dash of sauce (Worcestershire, Teriyaki, or Oyster)

Method

Preheat oven to 180°C (360°F)
Scrub and boil potatoes with skin on
Drain and mash the potatoes
Season with salt and pepper
Chop the onion
Grate the carrots
Melt the onions in the oil with the garlic and ginger
Put in the meat and fry it until it is brown breaking it up as it cooks.
Add the carrots, sauce, and herbs, stir and cook a few moments
Season with salt and pepper
Grease a large ovenproof dish
Put the mixture into the dish and level it out.
Cover with the mashed potatoes
If you wish, you could make a pattern on top with a fork and put some dabs of butter on to help browning
Put in the oven until the potatoes are brown on top (about 20 minutes)

Tips

Serve with a salad of raw vegetables

Eat slowly, so you enjoy your food.
Remember your portion control

Spaghetti Bolognaise

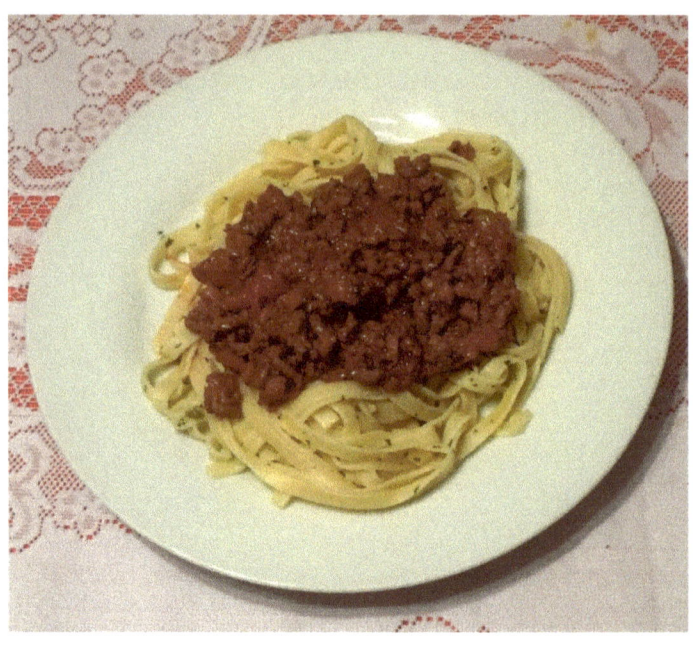

Ingredients (serves 4)

1 Packet of spaghetti (the choice is yours)
½ pound (500grams) of minced meat or, if you wish, you can buy about 4 large Chorizos, take the skin off, cut the chorizos up, and put them through a blender. It should look like mince after a minute or two.
1 large onion
2 tsp garlic or 4 or 5 pods of fresh garlic
1 can of diced tomatoes or 4 or 5 fresh tomatoes (diced)
250g Mushrooms (small cups or sliced)
1 cup of red wine
3 or 4 strips of bacon (cut the rind off)
1 bunch of parsley

Method
.
You will need two saucepans for this meal, one to boil the water for the spaghetti and another for cooking the Bolognese.
Start with slicing the onion, cook in a bit of oil, (olive oil if you have any in your Larder)
Add the minced meat fry it, turning the meat all the time.
When the meat starts turning brown add the bacon diced with the rind off.
Cook for a few minutes. Add the tomatoes and garlic. Stir it into the meat, add a bit of salt (be careful if you are using chorizos as they have got salt in them already).
If you wish to add about half a bottle of spaghetti sauce, do so; it will enhance the taste.
Cover the pan with a lid and cook the Bolognese on a low heat stirring from time to time until it is cooked completely.
Add mushrooms 10 minutes before end of cooking time
Bring a large pan of water to the boil put some salt into the water and insert the spaghetti into the pan making sure you get all of the spaghetti into the hot water.
Keep stirring the spaghetti, so it does not stick together.
Meanwhile, wash the bundle of parsley and chop it up to a very thin consistency.
When you think the spaghetti has been cooked, strain in a colander.
Put a knob of butter in the pan, put the chopped parsley in the pan, and stir it until it is mixed in with the butter, get the drained spaghetti and stir it into the parsley and butter mixture.

Tips
Eat slowly, so you enjoy your food.
Remember your portion control
A very good way to judge how much spaghetti to use for a person is to buy a gauge from your hardware shop.

Pork

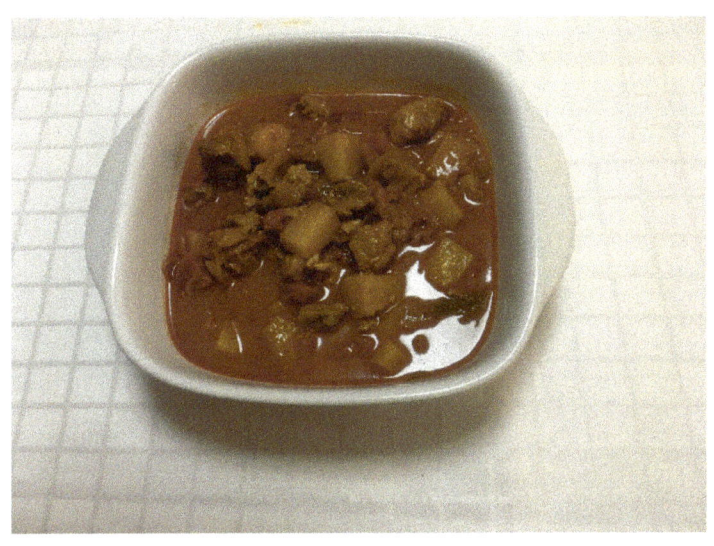

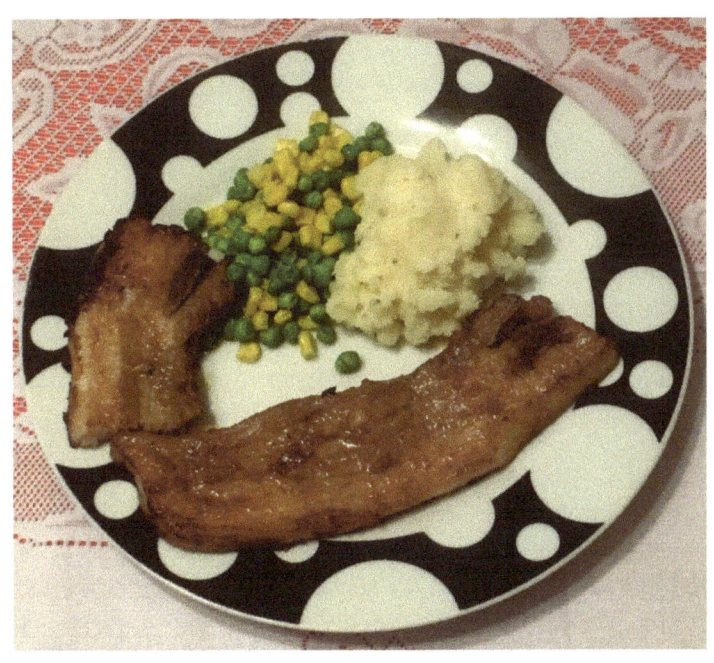

Belly of Pork and Pineapple Curry

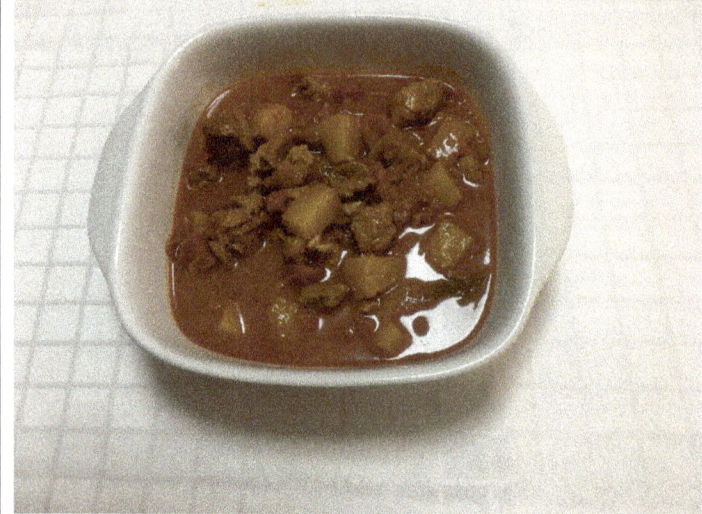

Ingredients (serves 4)

500g strips of belly of pork cut into cubes
1 large onion
3-4 heaped tbsp mild curry paste
1 can pineapple cubes or rings (if you buy the rings cut them into cubes)
A few curry leaves
1 small stem lemon grass
2 tbsp cooking oil
1 small piece of a pandanus leaf crushed and cut into small pieces
1 large can diced tomatoes or 5-7 large overripe tomatoes diced
1 small can coconut milk
½ to ¾ carton of beef stock
2 tsp garlic paste
2 tsp ginger paste

Method

Slice onion and fry in oil with diced belly of pork, stirring frequently, for a few minutes. Add curry leaves, lemon grass (crushed and cut into small pieces), pandanus leaf cut into small pieces, curry paste, Mix well. Add tomatoes. Stir well. Add the garlic paste and ginger paste. Stir. Add the coconut milk and beef stock and stir well.
Add the pineapple and ¼ of the juice
Cover and cook on a medium to low heat until the curry is cooked

Tips
This dish can be eaten with boiled rice, a stir-fry (see my recipe for the stir-fry) and devilled potatoes or potatoes in turmeric and coconut (see recipe).

Eat slowly, so you enjoy your food.
Remember your portion control

Belly of pork strips with mashed potato, steamed vegetables, and a side salad

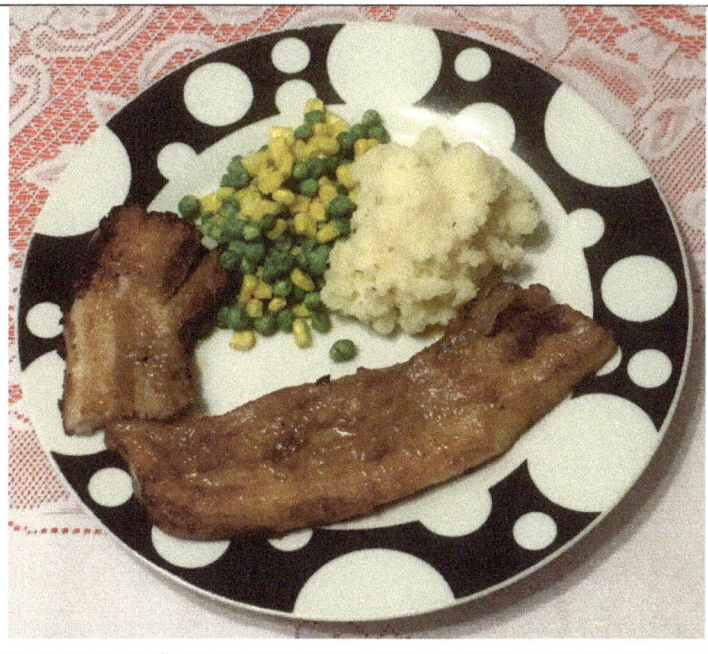

Ingredients (serves 4)
Pork Strips
1 strip of belly of pork per person especially for children – you may need two per adult)
A dash of garlic paste
A dash of ginger paste
Mixed dried herbs
A dash of Worcestershire sauce
A dash of soy sauce
Salt to taste (watch the salt, as the soy sauce is quite salty)
A dash of oil

Steamed Vegetables and side salad
Vegetables of your choice

Mashed Potato (see separate recipe)

Method
Pork strips
Mix all the ingredients with the pork strips
Place flat in a baking tray
Bake in a moderate oven 180°C (360°F) for 40 Minutes or until cooked through

Steamed Vegetables
Use any vegetables of your choice
Clean, peel, and cut up the vegetables
Steam in a steamer or colander over boiling water. Time will vary depending on the hardness of the vegetables and the size of the pieces.
Don't boil vegetables as all the nutrients are then thrown away with the water – this is not good!

Side Salad
Make a side salad with whatever vegetables you have. Try to eat as many raw vegetables as possible as they are very good for your digestion.

Tips

Eat slowly, so you enjoy your food.
Remember your portion control

Pork chop, baked potato, and steamed vegetables

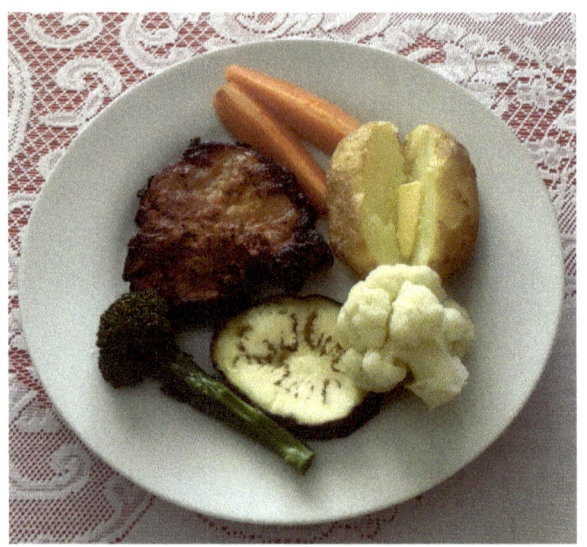

Ingredients (serves 4)

4 Pork chops
A dash of garlic paste
A dash of ginger paste
Mixed dried herbs
A dash of Worcestershire sauce
A dash of soy sauce
Salt to taste (watch the salt, as the soy sauce is quite salty)
A dash of oil

Steamed Vegetables (See separate recipe – page 34)

Baked Potato

Method

Snip the rind of the pork every 5mm (¼inch) with kitchen scissors. This lets the fat drain out and makes the rind into crackling.
Mix all the marinade ingredients and coat the pork chops on both sides but leave the rind dry.
Place flat in a baking tray
Bake in a Hot oven 220°C (430°F) for 10 Minutes then lower the heat to 180°C (360°F) for 30 minutes or until cooked through

Medium/small potatoes could be baked in the oven at the same time. If you want to keep the skins soft, you could wrap the potatoes in foil before cooking. Alternatively, you could bake them in a closed microwave dish with a little water for about 15 minutes for two medium potatoes. Check they are soft before opening them. Split and dab with butter.

Tips

Eat slowly, so you enjoy your food.
Remember your portion control

Lamb

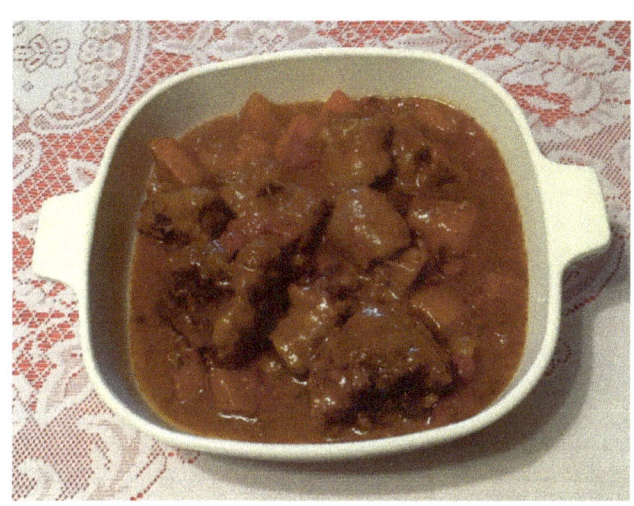

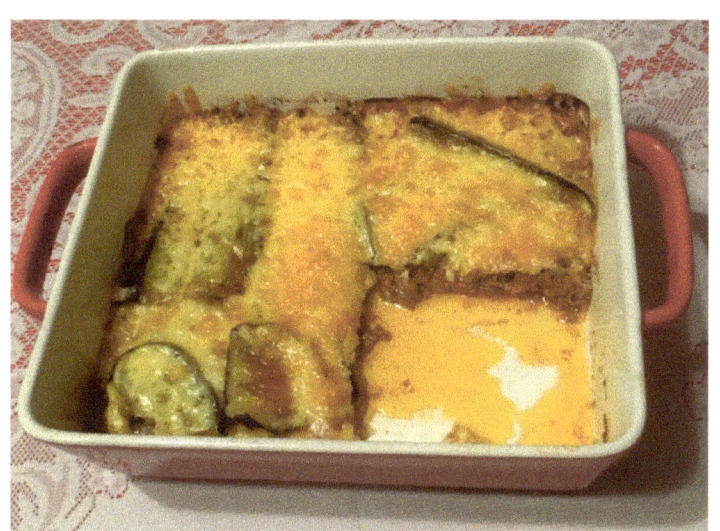

Lamb or Oxtail Stew

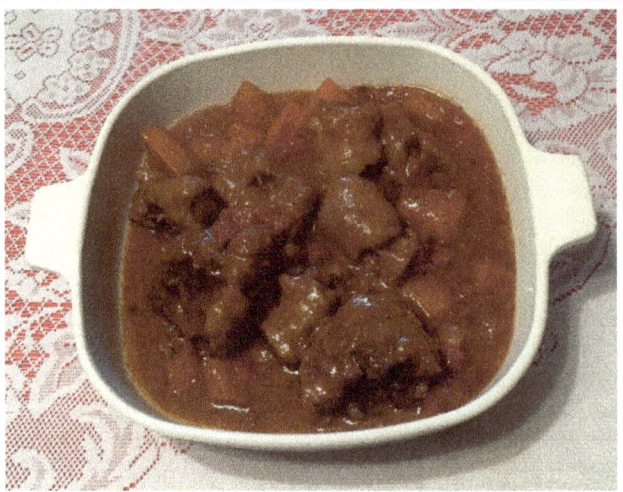

Ingredients (serves 8)

2kg (4lb) Stewing lamb or oxtail
1 large onion
2 tbsp oil
4 large carrots
4 large potatoes
1 large tin crushed tomatoes
Salt & pepper to taste
1 carton beef stock
1 tbsp soy sauce
2 tbsp Worcestershire sauce
2 tbsp cornflour

Method
Slice onion, fry in oil
Cut fat off the lamb. Fry lamb in a large pan.
Clean and wash carrots and potatoes. Cut into large cubes. Fry with the lamb
Add salt and pepper to taste. Add soy sauce and Worcestershire sauce,
In a bowl mix the cornflour with a little of the beef stock; make sure there are no lumps. Add cornflour mixture to the pan.
Add the can of tomatoes. Pour in the rest of the beef stock and stir well.
Make sure there is enough stock to cover everything.
Cook on a low heat. This will take a few hours as it is best if it is slow cooked. The meat should be very soft to the touch whether it is lamb or oxtail.

Tips
This recipe can be either lamb or oxtail stew.
It has to be slow-cooked, so I suggest cooking it the day before and keeping in the fridge overnight.
Serve with boiled rice and a side salad

Eat slowly, so you enjoy your food.
Remember your portion control

Moussaka

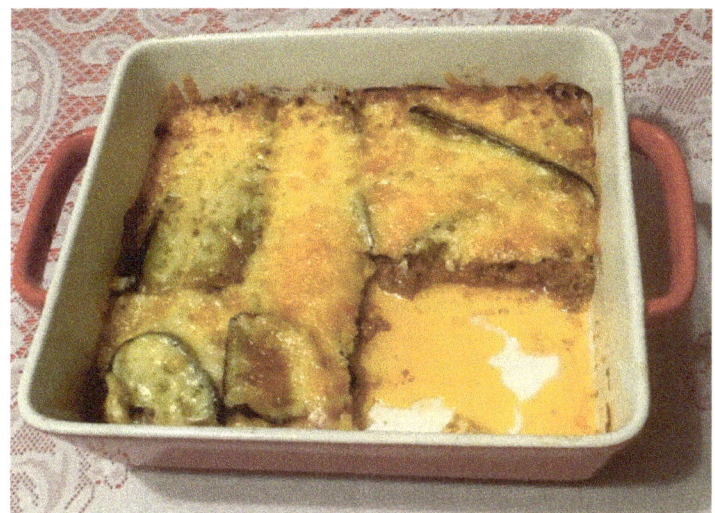

Ingredients (serves 4)
1 large and one medium sized eggplant

For the meat sauce
500g (1lb) minced beef or minced lamb
Oil for frying
2 large onions
1½ tsp minced garlic
½ cup of red wine
1 tbsp Worcestershire sauce
A dash of oyster sauce
4 large fresh tomatoes or 1 tin diced tomatoes
Salt
Pepper

For the cheese sauce
1 tbsp Butter
½ cup flour
2 cups Milk
1 cup grated cheddar cheese
1 tbsp grated parmesan cheese
Salt
Pepper

1 tbsp grated cheddar cheese

Method
Slice the eggplants lengthwise into ¼ inch (6mm) thick slices
Sprinkle the slices with salt and leave for at least 30 minutes, then rinse thoroughly and drain

Make the meat sauce:
Chop the onions and fry in a little oil until soft.
Add the garlic and fry for 30 seconds
Add the meat and fry until brown, breaking up the lumps and stirring
Add the wine and sauces
Add the chopped tomatoes
Season with salt and pepper
Simmer on a low heat for 20 minutes until the meat is cooked

Preheat oven to 180°C 360°F

Make the cheese sauce
Heat the milk until hot but not boiling   (Continued on next page)

In a saucepan melt the butter
Stir in the flour and mix thoroughly with the butter
Keep stirring and cook for about 5 minutes
Add a little of the hot milk stirring to make a smooth paste
Continue adding the milk and stirring
If there are any lumps, beat them out with a whisk
Add the cheeses and stir until dissolved
Season with salt and pepper
Remove from heat

Assemble the dish:
Use a greased pie-dish or casserole.
Put a layer of the eggplant to cover the bottom
Put a layer of the meat sauce
Another layer of eggplant
A layer of cheese sauce
Continue layering, ending with cheese sauce
Sprinkle the top with the grated cheese
(You can use breadcrumbs in this layer if you like)

Bake in the moderate oven for 30 minutes.
The eggplant should be cooked, and the cheese on top, starting to brown.

Tips

Eat slowly, so you enjoy your food.
Remember your portion control

Vegetables

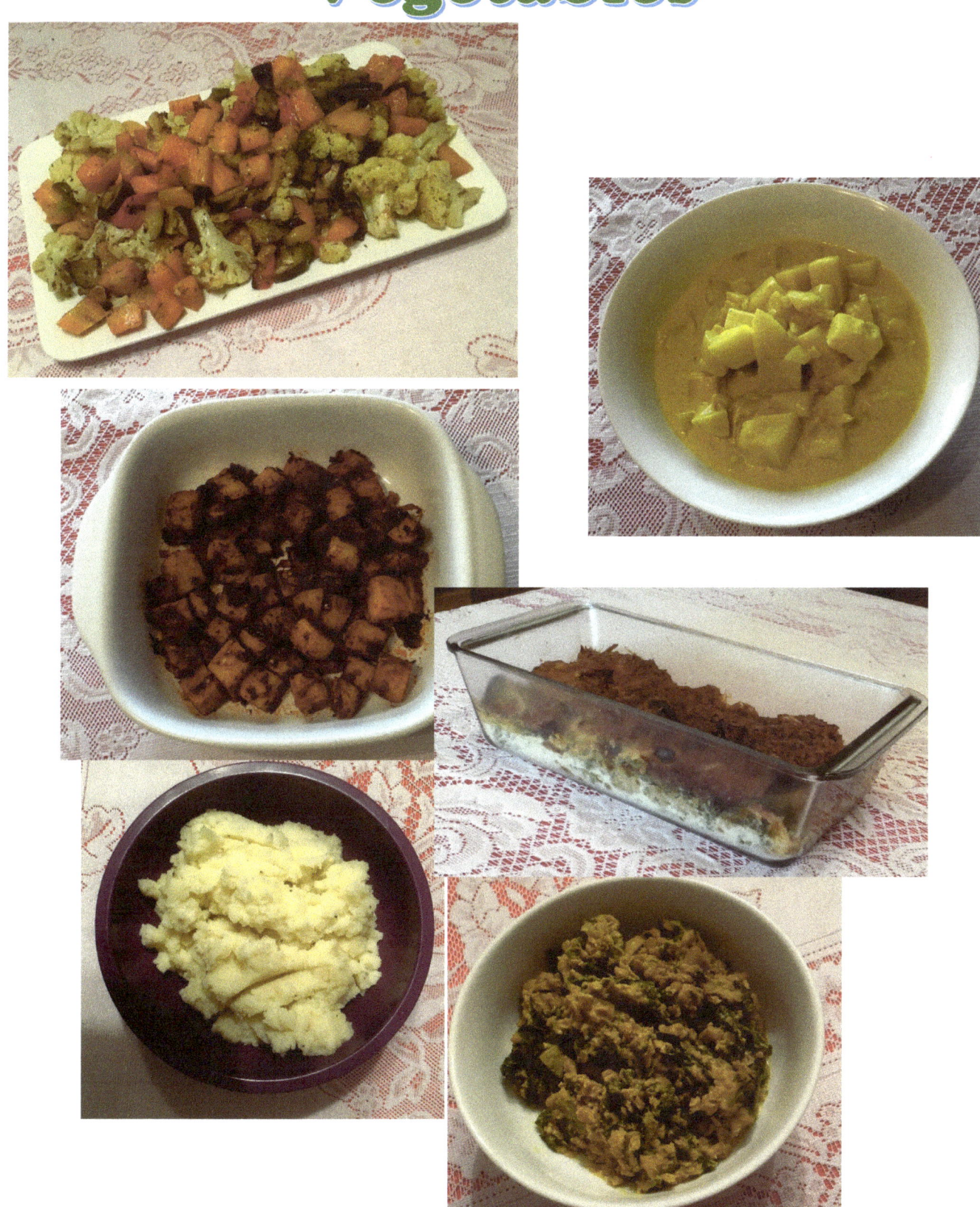

Yellow Potato in Turmeric & Coconut Sauce

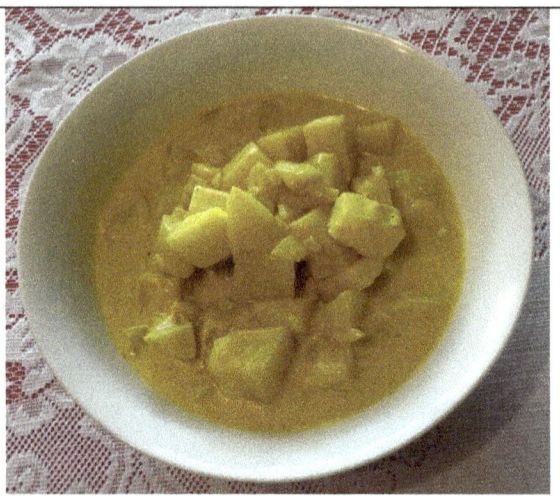

Ingredients (serves 4)
4 medium sized potatoes
I large onion
Salt to taste
1 heaped tsp Turmeric Powder
1 large can coconut milk or coconut cream
A little cow's milk
A few curry leaves
Oil for frying onion

Method
Wash and scrub potatoes thoroughly. If you wish you can leave the skins on as the skin is good roughage.
Cut potatoes into cubes. Boil in a large pan with plenty of water
While the potatoes are boiling, slice the onion. Add salt to taste. Fry the onions until they are cooked & transparent.
The potatoes should be cooked enough to be cooked but firm to the touch.
Drain the potatoes and add to the onion mix. Stir. Mix in the curry leaves, turmeric, and the coconut milk or coconut cream, Add the cow's milk.
Stir well and cook for a few minutes. Make sure the potatoes are cooked through. Don't cover the pan after you have added the milks as the contents will bubble up and overflow.

Tips
This makes an excellent accompaniment for a curry and can be eaten by people who do not like highly spiced (chilli hot) food. I serve it as an optional alternative to devilled potatoes.

Eat slowly, so you enjoy your food.
Remember your portion control

Devilled Potato

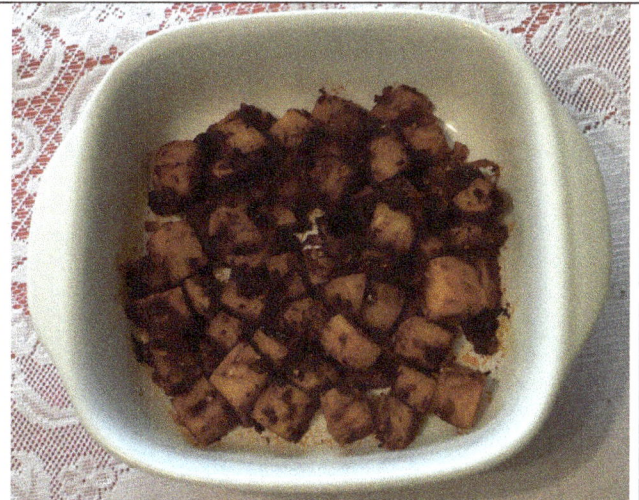

Ingredients (serves 4)
4 medium potatoes
1 large onion
Salt to taste
A few curry leaves
200 ml cooking oil
1 heaped tsp paprika (smoked or sweet)
Chilli powder or flakes to taste
Lemon Juice

Method
Wash and scrub potatoes thoroughly. If you wish you can leave the skins on as the skin is good roughage.
Cut potatoes into cubes. Boil in a large pan with plenty of water
While the potatoes are boiling, slice the onion. Add salt to taste. Fry the onions until they are cooked & transparent.
The potatoes should be cooked enough to be cooked but firm to the touch.
Drain the potatoes and add to the onion mix. Stir.
Mix in the curry leaves, paprika, and chilli, if used.
Stir well and cook for a few minutes. Make sure the potatoes are cooked through.
Add a squirt of lemon juice.

Tips

Eat slowly, so you enjoy your food.
Remember your portion control

This recipe is very similar to the Yellow Potato with Turmeric in Coconut Milk. I never serve devilled potato to children because it has, or could have, a lot of chilli flakes or chilli powder in it. I usually make enough of potato and divide it up, making some with turmeric and some to this recipe, depending on who is eating it and whether they like chilli-hot food

Mashed Potato

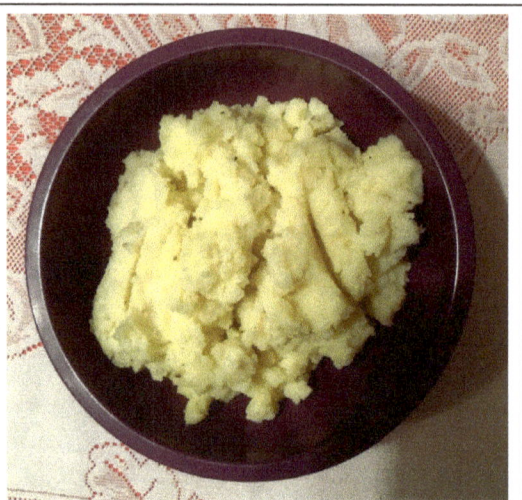

Ingredients (serves 4)

Potatoes (about 200g per person or more depending on appetite)
About 1tsp Butter per 200g potato
About ¼ cup Milk per 200g potato
Salt and pepper to taste
1 egg (optional)

Method
Peel potatoes and cut into chunks about 3cm across
Boil a pan of salted water and add the potatoes
Cook until soft when a knife is stuck into them (about 15-20 minutes). Some potatoes may start to break up when cooked.
Drain the potatoes and mash them with a potato masher or fork. It is important to mash them thoroughly before adding the butter and milk.
Add butter and mix it in.
Add milk until the mixture is smooth but not runny.
Season with salt and pepper.
If you like, you can add a beaten egg to make a stickier mash for coating or covering pies, etc.

Tips

Eat slowly, so you enjoy your food.
Remember your portion control

Mashed potato can be frozen. Other potato, (raw or boiled) goes grainy when frozen and never tastes right.

Roast Vegetables

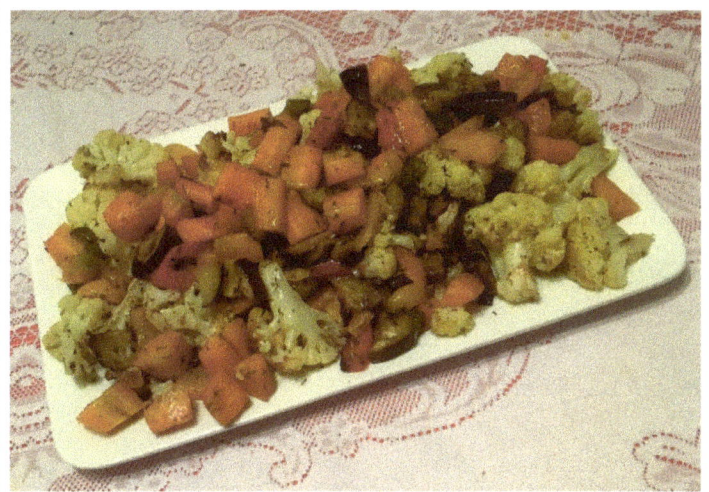

Ingredients (serves 4)

Use several different vegetables, aiming for different colours and textures as well as different tastes. This makes the dish interesting, beautiful and appetising as well as being healthy.
I typically use pumpkin, cauliflower, broccoli, eggplant (aubergine), carrots, and peppers. You can also include others depending on what is available.
Mixed dried herbs.
Salt to taste

Method
Wash all the vegetables.
Peel as required
Cut the vegetables up into convenient pieces. Aim for similar sizes.
With hard vegetables such as pumpkin and carrots, par-boil them before roasting.
Line an oven tray with foil and put a little cooking oil on it. Spread it to grease the foil and reduce sticking.
Put all the vegetables on the foil, spreading them out as much as possible.
Sprinkle with oil, mixed dried herbs and a little salt.
Bake in a moderate oven (180°C 360°F) for about 30 minutes until they start browning on top.

Tips

Eat slowly, so you enjoy your food.
Remember your portion control

Steamed Vegetables

Steaming vegetables is the best way to cook them unless you eat them raw. Never boil vegetables, as all the goodness is thrown away with the water.

Try to have three different vegetables (steamed) with your evening meal and salad with your lunch.

Enjoy your meals

Tips

Eat slowly, so you enjoy your food.
Remember your portion control

Vegetable bake with cheese

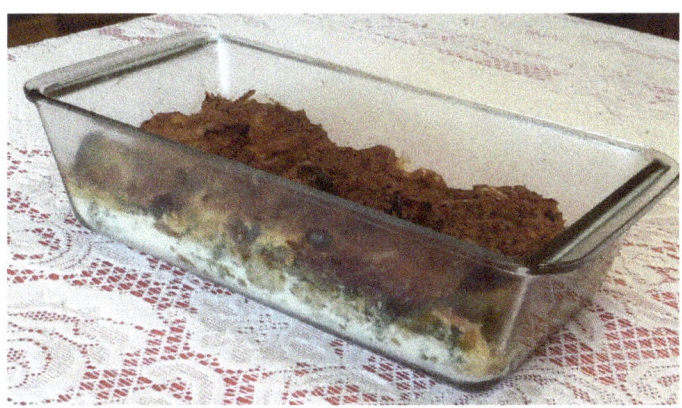

Ingredients (serves 4)

1 potato per person
Broccoli
Eggplant (Aubergine)
½ cup Grated cheese
¼ cup milk
1 egg
Salt and pepper to taste
Other vegetables as available

Method

Boil potatoes, slice and arrange in the bottom of a greased oven-proof dish.
Arrange a few broccoli florets and slices of eggplant
In a separate bowl, mix the cheese, milk, egg and season with salt and pepper.
Pour cheese mixture over the vegetables
Bake in the centre of the oven for 20 minutes or until the vegetables are cooked, and the cheese has melted through.

Tips

Eat slowly, so you enjoy your food.
Remember your portion control

Lentils with Spinach

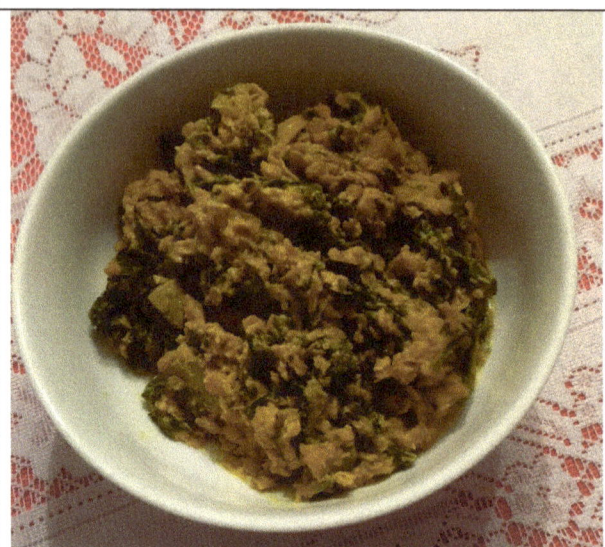

Ingredients (serves 4)

1 cup lentils (use red lentils)
1 medium onion
1 tsp Turmeric
¼ cup Milk or small tin of coconut milk
100g Spinach (Optional)
Salt

Method

Wash the lentils 2 or 3 times and strain it through a strainer.
Wash the spinach thoroughly
In a saucepan, cover the lentils with water and cook on a medium heat on top of your cooker. Keep an eye on the lentils as they will boil over if the flame is too high.
In a separate pan fry the onions and turmeric
When the lentils are soft, drain them and put them into the onion mixture
Add the milk
Add the spinach and stir
Continue to cook for 2 minutes
Season with salt to taste.

Tips

Eat slowly, so you enjoy your food.
Remember your portion control

Lentils go off very quickly after cooking so put them in the fridge after your meal.

Salads

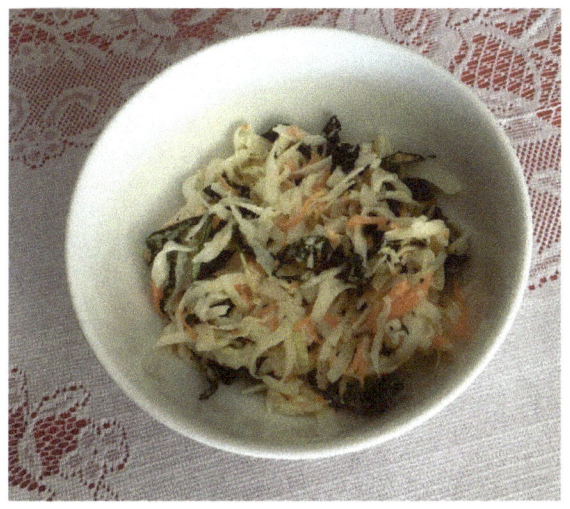
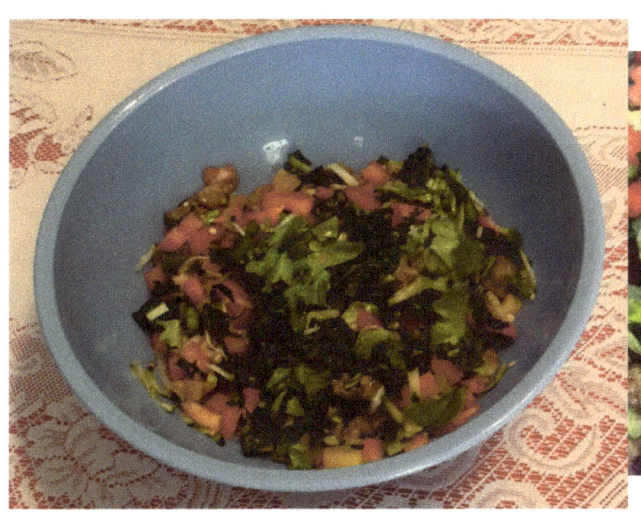
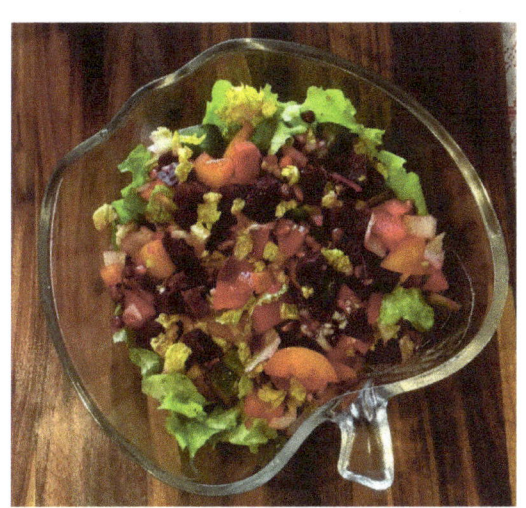
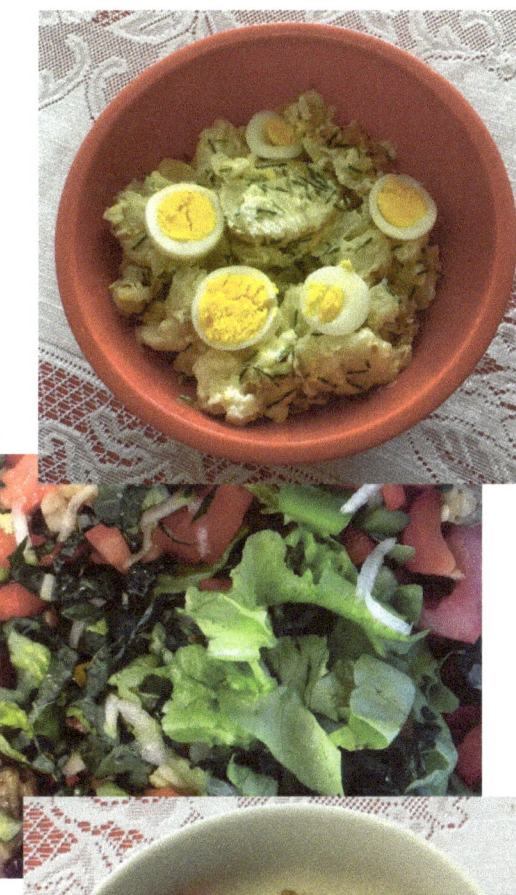
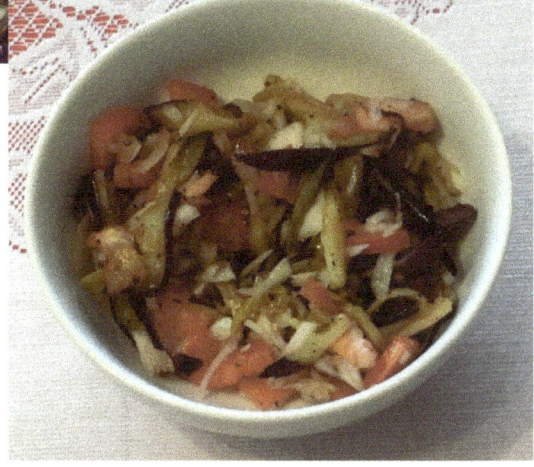

Coleslaw

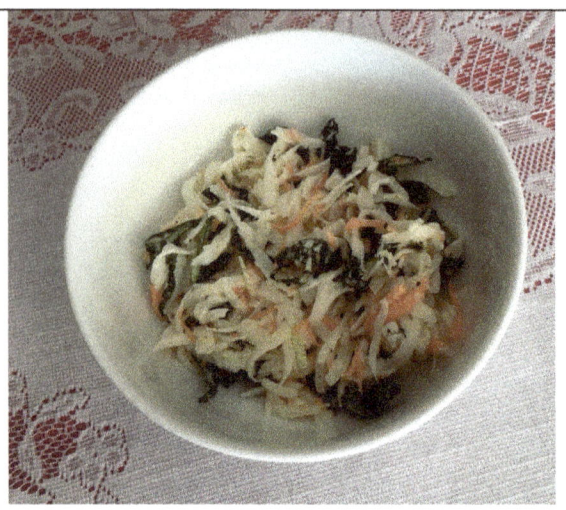

Ingredients (serves 4)

1 large carrot
¼ green or white cabbage
¼ Red cabbage
½ onion
1 tbsp lemon juice
2 tsp runny honey
¼ tsp mustard
1 small clove garlic
Salt
Pepper
½ cup sunflower or rice bran oil

Method
Finely grate the carrot
Shred the cabbage (I use a potato peeler to do this).
Finely grate the onion
Mix together in a bowl
In a separate small bowl mix the lemon juice and honey thoroughly
Crush the garlic (it is better for this purpose to crush the fresh garlic rather than use bottled garlic)
Add the mustard and garlic to the lemon and honey
Season with salt and pepper
Beat in the oil a little at a time until you have an evenly mixed dressing
Mix the dressing with the coleslaw

Tips

Eat slowly, so you enjoy your food.
Remember your portion control

You can try adding other shredded vegetables (for example Brussels Sprouts) to this coleslaw.

Potato Salad with Hard-boiled Eggs and Chives

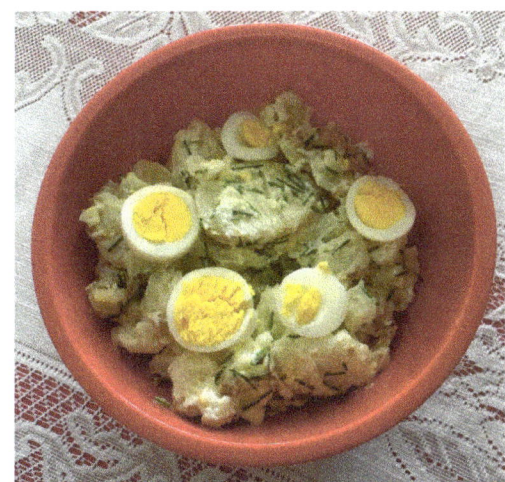

Ingredients (serves 4)

6 small potatoes (preferably a waxy variety)
1 tsp finely chopped onion
1 bunch chives
3 eggs
½ cup mayonnaise
2 tsp lemon juice
1 tsp honey
Salt

Method
Scrub the potatoes if they are thin-skinned, peel if thick-skinned.
Boil the potatoes until they are lightly cooked. You should be able to push a knife in easily, but they should not be overcooked to the point where they start breaking up.
Cut the potatoes across into slices.
Hard boil the eggs and peel
Chop two of the eggs coarsely and slice one.
Cut up the chives (easiest with scissors)
Mix the mayonnaise, honey and lemon. Beat thoroughly.
Gently mix the potato slices, chopped egg, mayonnaise, chives and a little salt. Try not to break the potatoes up.
Arrange the salad in a serving bowl and top with the sliced egg.

Tips

Eat slowly, so you enjoy your food.
Remember your portion control

Raw Vegetable Salad

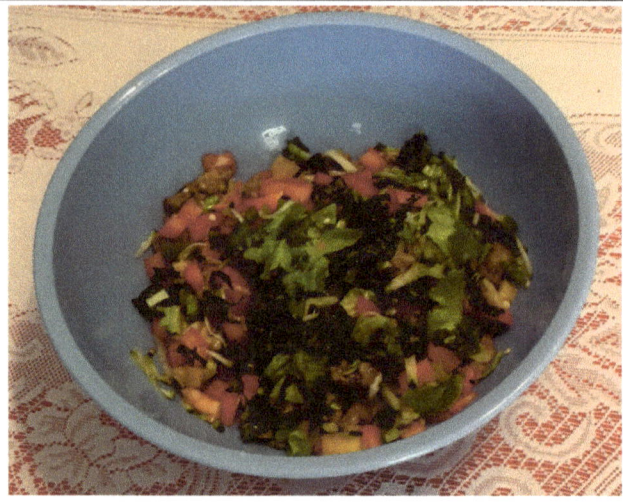

Ingredients (serves 4)

Cauliflower
Broccoli
Lettuce
Peppers (any colour or a mixture of the three colours)
Zucchini (Courgettes)
Spinach
Sprinkle of oil
Dried mixed herbs

Method

Wash the vegetables and cut up.
The zucchini can be grated
Add a sprinkling of olive oil and mixed herbs
Mix all together.

Tips

This raw salad is very good for you and tastes delicious.
Eat slowly, so you enjoy your food.
Remember your portion control
You can use any vegetable that can be eaten raw or include cooked vegetables like beetroot.

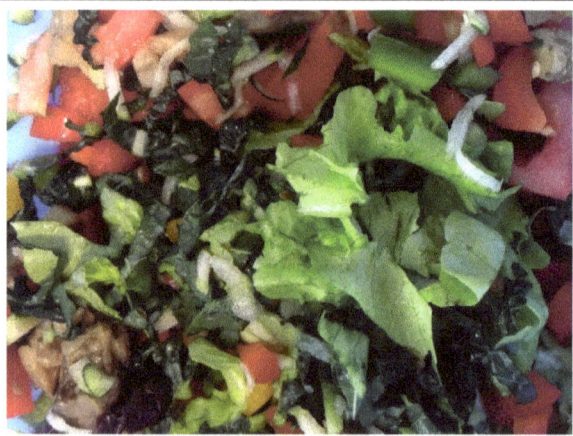

More detail of the salad

Eggplant Salad

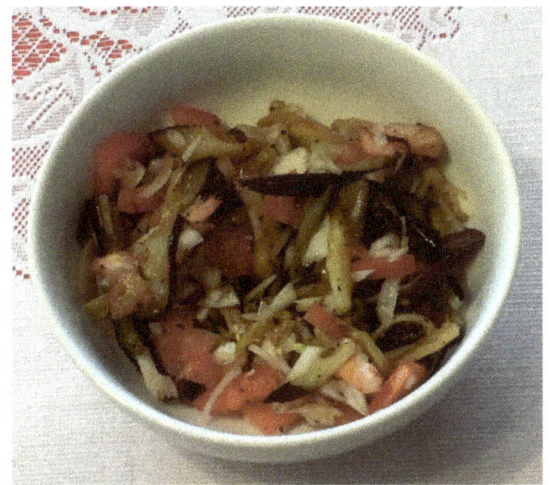

Ingredients (serves 4)

1 Large eggplant (aubergine)
1 large or 2 medium onions
A dash of lemon juice
¾ cup of oil
Salt and pepper to taste
2 tbsp dried shallots (crushed)
2 large ripe tomatoes

Method

Slice eggplant very thinly then cut into strips
Heat oil in a large pan. The oil needs to be very hot before you start frying.
Fry the eggplant until it turns soft and translucent
Drain the cooked eggplant on kitchen paper. Be careful of the hot oil left in the pan – put it away from any danger.
You can squeeze the eggplant a bit to get oil out.
Slice the onions thinly
Mix eggplant, and onions with sliced or diced tomatoes.
Add salt and pepper to taste and lemon juice
Mix everything together. Enjoy this lovely salad.

Tips

Eat slowly, so you enjoy your food.
Remember your portion control

Colourful Salad

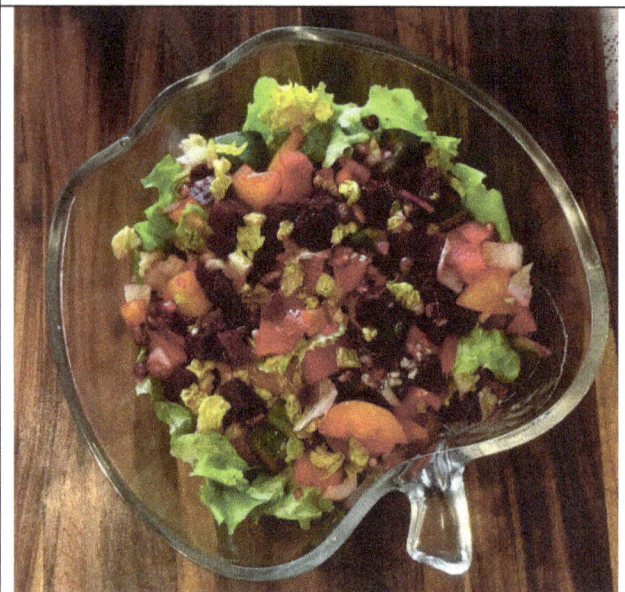

Ingredients (serves 4)

Light green curly leaved lettuce
Red, green and yellow peppers
Red and yellow grape tomatoes
1 pomegranate
Cooked beetroot
Salt
1 tbsp Lemon Juice
1 tsp Honey
¼ tsp mixed mustard
Sunflower oil or light flavoured olive oil
Salt to taste

Method

Wash all the vegetables
Cut the pomegranate in half and hit with a heavy spoon or the back of a knife over a bowl to get the seeds out and separate them. Pick out the white pith.
Arrange lettuce in the bottom of a serving bowl
In a small bowl mix the lemon juice and honey with the mustard. Beat with a fork. Gradually beat in the oil a little at a time. Add salt.
Mix the dressing with the chopped vegetables and the pomegranate seeds. Put them on the lettuce leaves.

Tips

Eat slowly, so you enjoy your food.
Remember your portion control

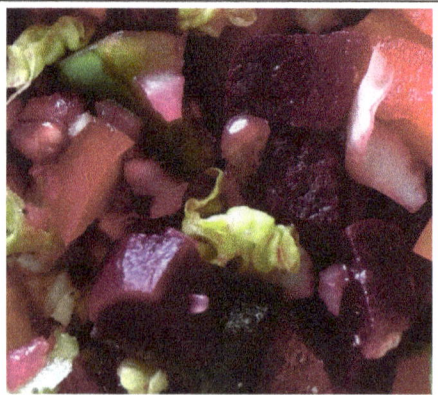

Detail of the salad. Note the pomegranate segment, glowing in the centre.

Rice

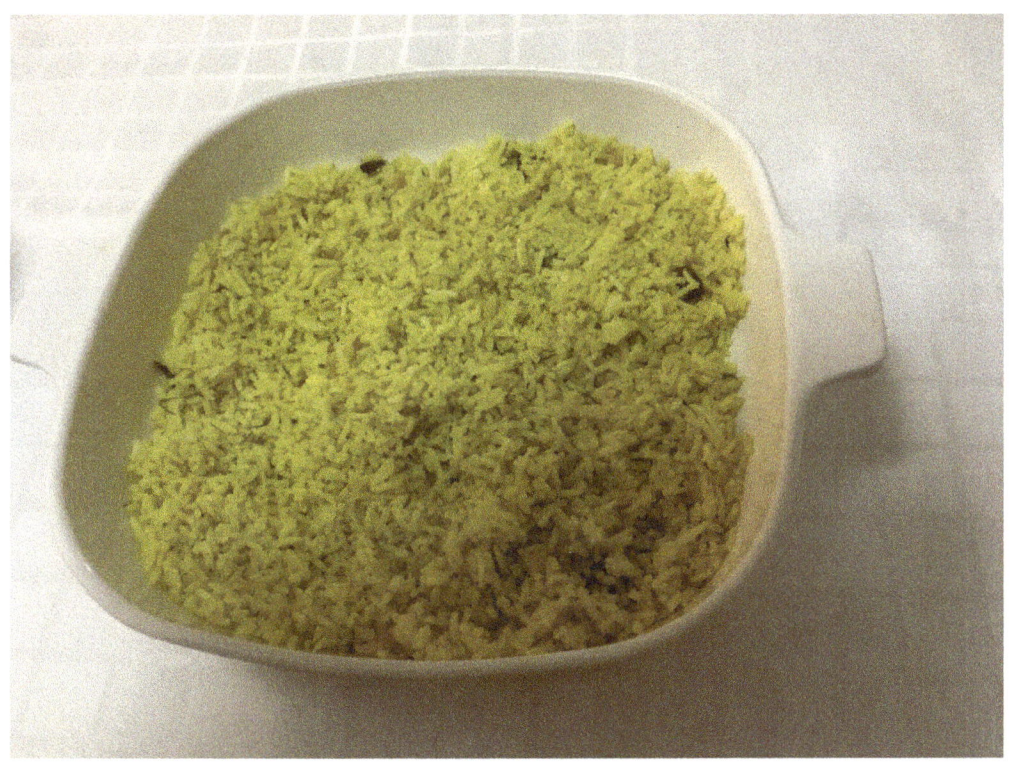

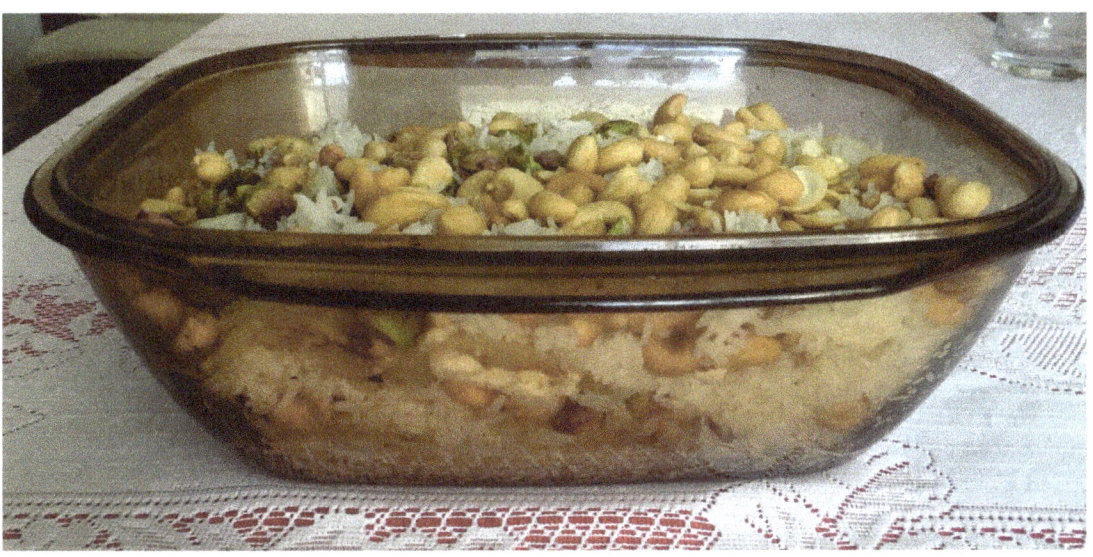

About Rice

Rice is a grain. There are many varieties used for food all over the world. It is high in carbohydrates (mainly starch) but does not have any gluten.

The rice I use most is white **basmati** rice. This rice has a distinct but mild flavour. It is a long-grained rice and, provided it is not overcooked, the grains separate well after cooking, making it light and fluffy. It is the best type to use for curries and stews or stir frying.

Jasmine or Glutinous rice is another white rice. It produces a lot of loose starch when cooked making it sticky. This makes it ideal when there is a need for the rice to stick together in a lump, as in sushi. It is used a lot in Japanese cooking.

Short grained rice takes a bit longer to cook and absorbs a larger proportion of liquid. This rice is mostly used for puddings, where it is baked in milk and swells to a gelatinous state by absorbing the liquid.

Brown rice has not had the husks removed. It has a light brown appearance when cooked and retains a springy, almost rubbery, consistency. It takes much longer to cook, and the grains remain separate. Some people like to eat it with curries. As the husks are not removed, it is higher in fibre than white rice.

Wild Rice also has its husks. The husks are black, and the grains are much longer than other rices. It also needs extra cooking time. Sometimes, people mix a little wild rice with white rice, mainly for the appearance of the contrasting black and white grains.

Cooking Rice

With white, long grain rice such as basmati, there are two main cooking methods.

Method 1: Absorption method

Wash the rice well until the water runs clear. Depending on the quality of your rice you may need to pick it over to remove any stones or other impurities. Drain the rice. Measure the rice into a large saucepan and add about 1¼ time as much water as rice. You have to experiment with this as it depends on the particular rice you are using and how long it has been kept. Add salt to taste, about ¼ tsp per cup of rice. Bring the rice to the boil, Lower the heat right down, so it is just simmering, put the lid on and until all the water is absorbed (about 11 minutes). You will see the rice absorbs all the water and holes start to appear in the surface. Test the rice and cook a little longer if needed. When the rice is cooked, remove it from the heat and stir with a large fork to separate the grains and fluff it up.

Method 2

After washing the rice, put the required quantity in a large pan with plenty of boiling salted water. Boil until the rice is cooked (about 11 minutes) then strain in a wire sieve. Rinse, first in cold running water to remove the starch, and then pour clear, boiling, water over it to reheat it.

Rice Cookers

These cook by the absorption method and make the process a bit easier.

Brown Rice is washed and then boiled in salted water for about 30 minutes until cooked. It does not need rinsing after cooking as it does not release much starch.

Yellow Rice

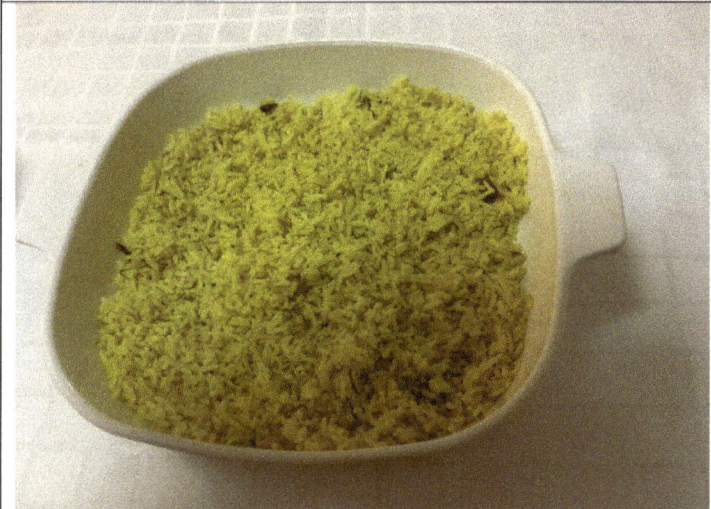

Ingredients (serves 4)

2 cups basmati rice
2½ cups water
1 tsp ground turmeric
salt

Method

I usually use a rice cooker. I will give you the recipes for both methods. First the rice cooker method.
I use Basmati rice as it is so easy to cook and really tasty.
The rice cooker comes with a measuring cup. Use 1 cup of rice per adult person and ½ cup for children.
Wash the rice until the water runs clear. Remember how many cups of raw rice you are about to cook.
In a frying pan, slice an onion, add salt, to taste, add a heaped teaspoon of turmeric powder and stir in the rice. If you can lay your hands on a few curry leaves and a piece of pandanus leaf, cut the pandanus leaf into small pieces and add them to the rice mixture.
Transfer the rice mixture into the rice cooker and put enough water to cover and go to the number of cups mark on the rice cooker. For example, if you used 4 cups of dry rice, put water up to the 4 cup mark on the rice cooker. I usually add a bit more water. Put the lid on and switch the rice cooker to "Cook". Leave it to cook, and when it is ready it will switch itself to "Keep warm". Enjoy your meal.

Absorption method
Prepare the rice mixture as above. Put it in a large pan with one and a quarter cups of water for each cup of dry rice used. Bring the rice to the boil, Lower the heat right down, so it is just simmering, put the lid on and until all the water is absorbed (about 11 minutes). You will see the rice absorbs all the water and holes start to appear in the surface. Test the rice and cook a little longer if needed. When the rice is cooked, remove it from the heat and stir with a large fork to separate the grains and fluff it up.

Tips

Eat slowly, so you enjoy your food.
Remember your portion control

Stir Fried Rice and Vegetables

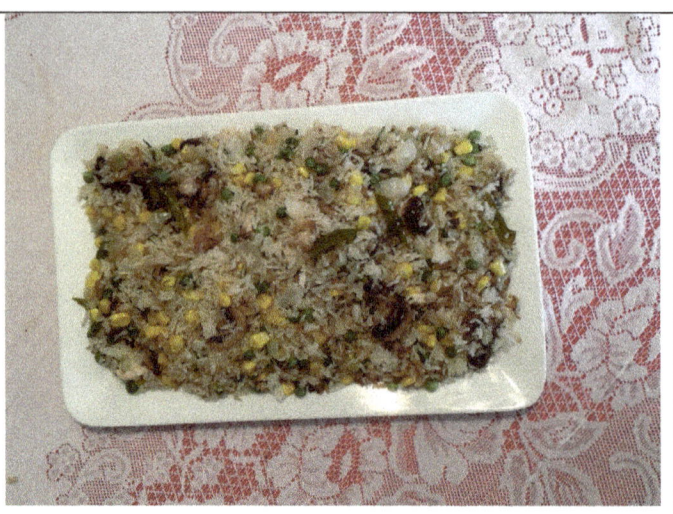

Ingredients (serves 4)

4 cups cooked rice
2 onions,
1/3 cup oil
curry leaves (if you can get any)
Diced bacon, (leave this out if you are vegetarian).
Cooked chicken (Ditto)
A cup of frozen corn kernels (cooked)
A cup of peas (cooked)
A dash of soy sauce
A dash of Worcestershire sauce

Method
Cook the rice your normal way.
Slice the onions. Fry in the oil.
Add the diced bacon
Add the diced chicken and curry leaves
Add cooked corn and cooked peas
Stir well. Add the soy and Worcestershire sauce
Stir well. Enjoy your meal.

Tips

Eat slowly, so you enjoy your food.
Remember your portion control

Growing time

Curry Leaf (Murraya koenigii)

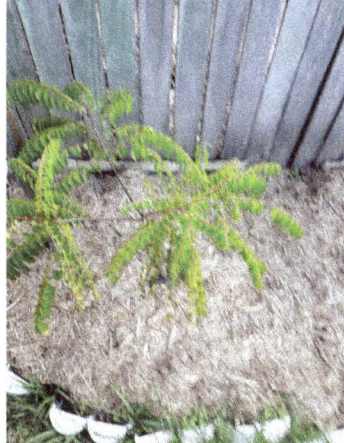

I use the leaves of the curry leaf tree quite frequently in my cooking. If you live in a cold country, don't worry as you can grow the curry leaf tree in a large pot indoors. Make sure you have a good compost and good nutrients in the soil. You can take the pot outside during the spring and summer season. Make sure you stand the pot in a saucer, indoors or outdoors. I also spread crushed eggshells around the base once in two months. This plant loves the calcium.

Lemon Grass (Cymbopogon citratus)

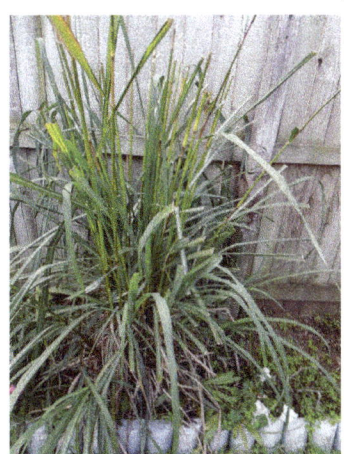

Lemon grass is a tall grass-like plant. The stalk is used for cooking. The stem has to be crushed with the heavy part of a large knife and then cut into very small pieces. It is used in all forms of cooking.

If you live in a cold country, you can grow this plant in a large pot indoors, and, like the curry leaf tree, take it out for the spring and summer. Stand the pot on a large saucer. The lemon grass has to be cut back frequently as it grows to quite a height. Remember only crush the stems to add to your cooking. Do not try to use the flower stems, as they are hard and woody, just the leaf stems.

Pandanus leaf (Pandanus latifolius, P. amaryllifolius)

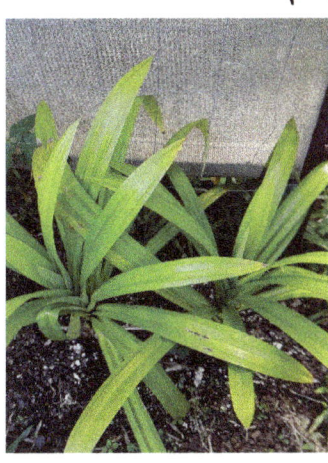

The pandanus has bright green leaves. Again, if you live in a cold country, this plant can be grown indoors, all the year through. Plant it in a large pot with lots of good compost. Once it grows to a certain height, if you look after the plant well, it will grow baby shoots. Wait until the baby plant is a reasonable height before you cut it off and plant it. Pandanus has a lovely aroma. Cut the leaf up into small pieces and add it to your cooking.

Last Words

Dear Reader

I hope you enjoyed my recipes and are producing good nutritious meals and saving money.

I would love to hear from you, and if you get in touch, I will let you know when I produce more books.

My website is CookingWithFewIngredients.com. The site has more recipes and tips for living well and keeping healthy.

You can contact me at Helen.Thomas@wise.works. If you do, I will reply.

Have a great time cooking and living healthily and cheaply.

Helen Thomas

www.ingramcontent.com/pod-product-compliance
Lightning Source LLC
Chambersburg PA
CBHW042015090526
44587CB00028B/4274